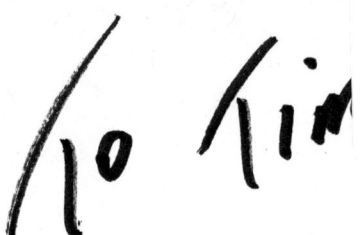

NEVER GIVE UP

THE MEANING OF MY LIFE
THE PAUL ROSEN STORY

Paul Rosen with **Roger Lajoie**

◆ FriesenPress

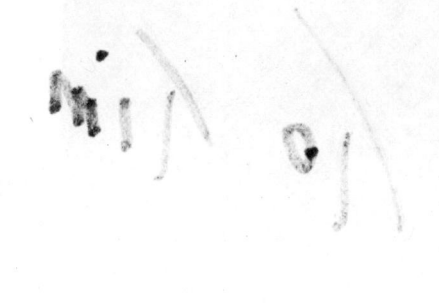

One Printers Way
Altona, MB R0G 0B0
Canada

www.friesenpress.com

Copyright © 2021 Paul Rosen and Roger Lajoie
First Edition — 2021

All rights reserved.

No part of this publication may be reproduced in any form, or by any means, electronic or mechanical, including photocopying, recording, or any information browsing, storage, or retrieval system, without permission in writing from FriesenPress.

ISBN
978-1-03-912499-8 (Hardcover)
978-1-03-912498-1 (Paperback)
978-1-03-912500-1 (eBook)

Biography & Autobiography, Personal Memoirs

Distributed to the trade by The Ingram Book Company

Table of Contents

Introduction
Chapter 1: Let's Talk 1
Chapter 2: Growing Up 5
Chapter 3: Working life 11
Chapter 4: Rehab woes 17
Chapter 5: Meeting Max 19
Chapter 6: Losing limb 25
Chapter 7: Sledge Hockey 29
Chapter 8: Team Canada 33
Chapter 9: PR man 37
Chapter 10: First Paralympics 41
Chapter 11: Funeral business 45
Chapter 12: Top goalie 49
Chapter 13: Coaching Canada 53
Chapter 14: Getting funded 55
Chapter 15: Max's fall 57
Chapter 16: Second Olympics 61
Chapter 17: Marriage ends 69
Chapter 18: Family tragedy 71
Chapter 19: Medal stolen 73
Chapter 20: Sitting volleyball 85
Chapter 21: SLED HEAD 89
Chapter 22: Darker times 93

Chapter 23: Vancouver Olympics 97
Chapter 24: Retirement time 107
Chapter 25: Road Hockey 111
Chapter 26: Broadcasting debut 115
Chapter 27: Jubilee Medal 119
Chapter 28: Another Olympics 123
Chapter 29: Downward spiral 127
Chapter 30: Fateful night 133
Chapter 31: Getting care 137
Chapter 32: Broadcasting again 143
Chapter 33: Gouche Live 151
Chapter 34: Battling COVID 153
Chapter 35: Four stories 157
Chapter 36: Life's meaning 165
About the Author

INTRODUCTION

"The meaning of my life is to help others find the meaning of theirs."
— Viktor Frankl

Never give up.

That's what Paul Rosen signs his photos with when he gives them out at his various public speaking engagements. That's three great words to leave people with for sure - just a fantastic message to give someone – NEVER GIVE UP!

Rosey told me he always wanted to write his memoirs but he never got around to it. I'm glad he never gave up on that goal, because here we are.

This is his story, as told by him and written by me. I wrote the autobiographies of legendary Canadian hockey player Paul Henderson and hockey executive Jimmy Devellano in the same vein. I really didn't expect to write another one frankly, but like I said, here we are.

Never Give Up…The Meaning of My Life. By Paul Rosen with Roger Lajoie…what a pleasure for me to be able to help Paul bring his story to life.

I had met Paul Rosen several times before this project and knew "of him" like many Canadians do, but I didn't really know him that well. So I interviewed Paul for many, many hours to get all the details of his fascinating life's journey. I watched games he played in and features about him on YouTube and elsewhere. I read numerous articles which featured Paul, some on his playing career and others on his time as a motivational speaker.

Rosey has lived quite a life and has overcome a great deal of adversity, as you will see in these pages. He has a lot of great stories and memories and his journey is very well worth documenting. It was really a privilege to do this with him.

Paul wanted to be candid in this book and he wanted to document his life honestly, especially the difficult parts of which there are many. But at the same time he made this clear to me – he didn't want to hurt anyone and write anything that could cause anybody any pain. He wanted to accept the responsibility for all of the pain he might have caused other people, but he didn't want anyone to feel bad themselves as a result of reading this. He does not have to worry about that.

What you will read in the following pages are his memoirs as told in his own words, through me. There is not a word in here that he did not approve of. He talked, I wrote and he approved. He has certainly lived a life worth writing about and this book carries an important message throughout – never give up.

Yet on January 30, 2019, Paul Rosen attempted to take his own life. Yet on other many occasions in his six decades on the planet, he experienced crippling depression and addiction that almost crushed him. Yet even while he used his enormous talents as a public speaker to encourage other people to live life to the fullest, he often found enormous difficulties in doing that himself.

He was like a lot of us. He didn't take his own advice.

If anyone ever talked to you the way Paul Rosen told me he often times talked to himself, Paul Rosen would likely punch you in the face! (OK he is too nice to do that, but he'd let you have it verbally for sure). There is nobody who has been more supportive and caring to other people than Rosey. You hear just one of his talks and you can see that is true…yet at times he found it hard give himself the same sort of compassion he was so good at giving to other people.

So, what is the meaning of all that then? What was the meaning of his suicide attempt? What is the meaning of Paul Rosen's entire life when all is said and done?

I think that's what Paul Rosen was trying to figure out for a long time, especially after that dark day in January 2019. He found his answer. It's in this book, so please read on.

Everything Paul Rosen has gone through in his life, all of his difficult times, do indeed have a meaning, especially the night he tried to end it. It is so clear now. I saw it right away once we started doing our interviews. By the time we were done he saw it too.

I am so happy about that.

NEVER GIVE UP

His story of overcoming adversity, of overcoming addictions, of overcoming his own demons, has a very important meaning. The meaning of this book and his life is – well I can't give that away in the introduction, can I now?

Thank you Paul for letting me help you write this book and find your answer. You are a good man sir.

Love you Rosey.

Never give up.

Roger Lajoie

September 1, 2021

CHAPTER 1

LET'S TALK

It was January 30, 2019. It was Bell Let's Talk Day, an initiative I had supported for many years.

Mental health issues had always been important to me, so I accepted an invitation to speak about overcoming adversity to a group of school kids. It always meant a lot to me to do those kinds of talks, and the kids I spoke to always seemed to enjoy them and get something out of them.

Being a motivational speaker was something I had been doing for more than a decade by then. I was a talker. I had done hundreds of these kind of events and this was just another one on the schedule.

This particular talk went especially well. I spoke for about a half an hour and got a great reception from the kids. There was lots of clapping, lots of smiles, and several came up to me at the end of my talk and told me how much it had meant to them.

I often got a positive reaction and this one was even better than most.

"Rosey, you're the best!" one of the kids said to me. He had a huge smile on his face. I obviously said some things that really resonated with him.

It always brings a tear to my eye when I see someone react so positively to what I have to say about overcoming adversity and never giving up on life. That's my primary message at most of the talks I do, and that was the message I gave on this day.

There were lots of high fives and slaps on the back all around. There were lots of great individual moments with the kids. There were lots of hugs…and a few tears of joy too.

The teachers who had invited me to speak at their school thanked me profusely. It had always amazed me how positively my talks were received, whether they be in a school or a business or wherever. I must have shook hundreds of hands that morning and exchanged dozens of hugs.

I gave them a good talk. I really did…and they appreciated me.

I thanked everyone for such a great reception and I left after being there for about an hour and a half to drive back home to the tiny little apartment I had at that time in downtown Toronto. Chalk up another talk on never giving up into the books for the much loved Paul Rosen.

As I drove, I started thinking. I started thinking about what I was going to do for the rest of the day. I started planning every detail.

By the time I arrived at my apartment, I had everything all worked out in my mind. I knew just what I was going to do and how I was going to do it.

I was going to kill myself that night.

◘ ◘ ◘

I don't remember much about that entire month of January 2019 to be truthful. In a three week span that month, all kinds of things happened to me and most of them were really bad.

On December 13 of the previous year, I had hip replacement surgery and it had been an ordeal. Over Christmas and New Year's I was basically stuck in a wheelchair most of the time, not even bothering to put my artificial leg on. On most days I was just in bed all day, doing no therapy, and living in constant pain.

I was depressed big time. Basically the only time I ever left my apartment during that month was to go and do a talk somewhere, like the one I did on the morning of January 30. I was going to talk to some students about what great futures they'd have if they never quit, but I didn't really see any future for myself.

My hip was killing me. I was taking pain killers like they were candy. For years I had been addicted to narcotics and alcohol and was abusing them both pretty badly, but even that no longer dulled the pain – both the emotional pain and physical pain – that I was constantly feeling.

I had thought of killing myself many times over the years, but had always kept those thoughts to myself. It wouldn't do my motivational speaking career much good if people knew I was suicidal a lot of the time. That would be bad for business.

What had stopped me from doing more than just thinking about suicide were my three kids. The thought of the pain they would have if I ever did it stopped me. The thought of the pain of the many people I had encouraged never to give up would have also made me reconsider. How would all the people my talks had helped feel if they heard that Paul Rosen had killed himself, I would often wonder to myself.

I didn't stay alive for me. I stayed alive for them.

I wasn't thinking about other people's feelings that night though. I was only thinking about the pain I was suffering. The pain was just too much.

"Everybody loves Rosey" I thought to myself. "Everybody thinks I am king shit."

But what I really felt like was a piece of shit. I felt worthless. I told myself I was done.

I saw only one way out of my pain on the night of January 30, and that was to kill myself. After years of thinking about suicide, I had decided that tonight was the night I would do it…just hours after I had talked to those great kids.

❂ ❂ ❂

I made myself something to eat at around 4:30. I cried a lot. I just hated myself. Deep down I guess I wanted to convince myself not to do it, but I felt I really had to do it now. I just felt I was done, tired of living a lie, and tired of all the physical and emotional pain that had plagued me for years.

I lay down and watched some sports on TV, which is basically how I had spent most of my days since the hip replacement surgery. There was a documentary on about Rick Rypien, the NHL player who had killed himself. It was Bell Let's Talk Day, so I guess that's why they were airing that particular show. How ironic.

After I ate I called my kids one final time. I didn't let on what I was going to do; I just wanted to hear their voices before I did it. Even though my kids were the reason I had never attempted suicide before, I could not escape the thought that I was a loser and that the world would be better off without me. I knew it would hurt them terribly but I was too far gone to have that stop me this time.

I then wrote a letter to them. It was a suicide note. I wanted to tell them how much I loved them one more time and try to explain what I had done.

After that…I made sure I was nice and cleaned up. Here's the reason why that was so important for me on that day.

For six years earlier in my life I had worked for Benjamin's Funeral Homes, a job that I really enjoyed. It was that experience that led me to do what I did next – I took a bath and put on fresh underwear and a clean pair of shorts.

I wanted to be mindful and considerate towards whoever picked me up when it was discovered what I had done. Part of my duties at Benjamin's was to transport dead bodies to the morgue, so I knew how tough a job that was at the best of times. I just wanted to make sure I was not a mess for them to handle. I had to deal with some very disturbing things during my time doing that kind of work, and I didn't want to be dirty and disgusting for the people who would come and pick me up.

I took my bottle of Oxycodone pills out (known as poor man's heroin). I counted the pills I had left; there were 35 of them. I thought that was more than enough to do the trick.

I divided them into three piles of 10, 10 and 15 pills. I took the first 10, had some water, took the next 10, had more water, and then took the final pile of 15, again with lots of water.

I then got into bed and put the covers up, closing my eyes. The note was clearly visible on a table near the door and I was clean and ready.

I was ready to go away, to fall asleep, and to never wake up again.

Paul Rosen was ready to do what he had told everyone else NOT to do for so long.

I gave up.

CHAPTER 2

GROWING UP

I came into the world on April 26, 1960 at Toronto's Old Mount Sinai Hospital. I weighed in at just under 10 pounds, the second of four children that Clarice and Ronald Rosen had. Reports are that I immediately started talking.

My brother Steven was four years old when I arrived. My sister Gail (who I get my caring and giving side from without question), was born two years later, and my other brother Brian came along on July 9, 1967. Brian died just seven days after he was born from spinal meningitis, rest his sweet soul.

My Dad was a truck driver with Crawford Sand and Gravel. We were a working class family in every sense of the word. We didn't have a lot of material possessions, but we had enough to get by. There were a lot of families like that back in the 1960s in our neighborhood. We struggled but we survived. My parents were good people.

We lived for a while on Grand Ravine Avenue, just off Keele between Finch and Sheppard, in Toronto. I went to Stylecroft Public School and almost from the start of my life, became a bit of a troublemaker.

There were a lot of reasons why I was, but probably the biggest was that right from the start, I hated school. I hated to read and I hated to write and for the first few years of anybody's school career, that's mostly what you do – read and write.

I wasn't very good at either reading or writing. When you have a literacy problem like I had, you tend to gravitate to becoming a class clown and I guess that was what I became at school. Becoming the focus of attention for my outlandish behavior took the focus off my inability to learn properly.

I got punished a lot because of the way I acted. In all honesty, my Dad beat the daylights out of me sometimes. It was a different world back then, and he certainly wasn't the only dad that would do that to his son, but when I was bad at school or at home he would really let me have it.

Let me be clear here – I don't blame him my father was a product of his times. I guess in many ways so am I.

I'd try so hard to have a great week. If I wasn't in any trouble, my Dad would take me for a drive in the truck he drove and I'd get to blow the horn. Some of my fondest memories with my dad are of those times when it was just him and me, together in that truck driving around. I only mention the beatings I got because I am going to be totally honest with everything in this book; it happened. He beat me. But I loved my Dad then and I love him to this day.

Most of my problems stemmed from the times when I was actually at school. I was a troublemaker for sure; I did a lot of dumb things at school, so I earned many of those punishments. In that era you weren't sent to a corner for some quiet time, you got hit. That's just the way it was.

I don't fault my Dad for all this. We didn't have a lot of money but thanks to him we had a decent life at home. It's not that we were really lacking anything. But for whatever reason, I just couldn't stay out of trouble growing up. I did a lot of bad things, just plain dumb stuff – one time I even cut one of the power lines that went to the nearby synagogue, putting it in darkness for several hours. I was 12 years old at the time, it was just a stupid prank done by a stupid punk.

My parents dealt with me the best they could. As for the schools I was in? The schools didn't really care what I was up to frankly. At that time they didn't really have the processes in place to handle kids like me, and the even the school's principal didn't care. They were just overwhelmed with everything they had to do with scant resources in those days. They didn't have time to deal properly with troublemakers like me.

I was funny, a bit of a charmer. My punk actions usually didn't hurt anybody, just myself. And I had one thing going for me that really saved my bacon with everybody in the school, especially the teachers.

I was a great athlete.

I played on every school team growing up. I was involved in just about every sport and I was good at them all. I mentioned that the principal didn't really care about my antics and there was a reason for that. He just wanted the school's teams to win championships, and I helped the school win more than a few with my athletic abilities. That's why they mostly left me alone when I acted up.

Playing sports was my solace during my school days. I was a miserable failure in the classroom, getting marks like 55 in History and 30 in Math, but I was a star outside of the classroom. That was good enough for me and I guess it was good enough for the schools I attended too.

By the time I made it into junior high school, at Eliah Junior High School, I was a total train wreck in the classroom. I even failed Grade 8 – twice! After I failed the second time, the school made a deal with my family that saw me get transferred to Northview High School. I was put in a class that was basically for dummies…there is no other way to put it.

Anybody who couldn't keep up in the regular classrooms was put together. That way we couldn't distract the rest of the kids who were there trying to learn.

That's just the way things were done back then. Schools didn't have the processes or the resources to handle kids who had literacy issues, or who were discipline problems in any way. The answer to those problem kids was to put them together in classes for slow learners. The other kids would call us "the retards" and make fun of the fact we weren't learning properly. That's hardly the right environment to encourage us to learn, but once you were assigned to that class that's just the way it was.

Let me make this clear however; I am not blaming the system at that time. I spent one year at Northview and regardless what class or program they put me in, I was never in class – period! Any chance I had at eventually being a good student was gone thanks to the fact that I was usually gone…as in not in attendance!

All I was interested in was sports. Sports were my entire life. I don't know how I graduated, but technically I did. I suspect my mother might have help cut a deal with the school just to get me out of there, and a lot of kids were just moved along through the system back in those days just to get them out the door and away from the other students.

I don't know for sure if that was the case with me, but I do know I have a high school diploma, which I got when I was 18 years old. I also know that I did virtually nothing to earn it.

The only thing I was good at in high school was playing sports. I was so good in fact, that I made the senior volleyball team when I was just in Grade 10. Making that team led to some great memories on the court – we had a great team – but some terrible memories off the court.

It was then that I became the victim of sexual assault at the hands of my female coach.

She was a teacher at the school and she was 39 years old. I was 17. She was absolutely stunning, and she took advantage of my youth and inexperience. She lived right across the street from the school, and it all started when she invited me back to her place one day after practice to talk about the team. She did a lot more that day than just talk.

This went on for months. I just couldn't bring myself to talk about it to anybody, mostly out of embarrassment. I was a male, she was a female, and I know the reaction I would have got. After a while I felt I had to say something to her at least – I told her we had to stop doing this. She would have no part of that however, and she was in a position of authority at the school so I just felt I had to stay quiet.

There were just a couple of guys on the team that knew what was going on, but they weren't going to say anything either. It controlled my day-to-day thoughts, and it became a massive reason why I behaved the way I did in school now that I look back on it – I was out of control in the classroom, a class clown – the abuse really did scar me emotionally.

I hadn't thought about her in years, but going through trauma counseling brought it all back. It made a bad situation for me at school all the more worse and I believe may have contributed to problems I had later on in life.

School life was just not for me. I was incapable of learning anything it seemed. But I was still an athlete, and a pretty good athlete at that. I was good enough to play hockey at a pretty high level, with the Thornhill Thunderbirds minor midget, midget and juvenile teams, for a couple of seasons, and I really loved that time away from school. I couldn't wait to get out of there and leaving school for good was nothing but a relief to me.

The hockey playing ability that I had turned out to serve me well later down the road. But that was still very much further down the road. And while hockey was the reason for a lot of my later success, my love of the game and playing the game as hard as I did would also be one of the main reasons I later lost my leg.

NEVER GIVE UP

So I was in trouble (of my own doing) a lot as a kid, but playing sports did keep me in shape. I was strong physically because of my involvement in sports, and I really loved playing them. It didn't hurt that I was pretty good at most of them either.

I never thought that I going to make a living out of playing hockey, but I was good enough to get some playing time with the Thornhill Thunderbirds as a right winger. I played a tough aggressive game and loved playing the sport. It was a real passion of mine.

Playing hockey and other sports didn't require me to read or write. All I had to do was play. And like a lot of other young kids my age, I played a lot of hockey and truly loved playing every minute for the Thunderbirds.

In May 1975 however, I suffered the first serious injury to my leg that would be the start of a long and painful process for me that continued throughout my life. I was skating down the right side during a game in my midget year and my right skate hit a rut in the ice.

I collapsed right away and knew it was serious. I suffered a fractured leg that ended my playing time for that season. It was a serious enough injury to also end any slim aspirations I might have had at ever doing more with my athletic ability than just being a recreational athlete.

Make no mistake about it; I knew I wasn't ever going to play in the National Hockey League or anything like that. However that first injury was just the start of a series of injuries to my leg that were going to plague me for the rest of my life.

Those injuries didn't stop me from playing men's league hockey, as I was a real stubborn son of a gun. About a year later, I'm playing in a men's hockey league game and I break that same leg again. The pain from the injury was horrible, but it wasn't as bad as the pain of not being able to play in our league's championship game because of the injury.

So I then did what is in retrospect one of the dumbest things I have ever done in my life. My leg was in a cast, but I took a hacksaw to that cast and cut the cast off so I could play in the final game. Talk about dumb!

I played that night and what a hero I was. I scored all three goals in a game that we won 3-2! But I had also taken a real risk at suffering some permanent damage to my leg just by trying to play, but that didn't matter to me at the time. All that mattered to me was playing hockey, and play I did, broken leg and all.

When I look back on that and reflect on how much a factor that decision to play that night could have played in my future health problems, I just shake my head. You'll read in these pages about some of the dumb things I've done in my life, and this is certainly at the top of the list.

I chose being a men's league hockey hero over staying healthy. It worked out great on that one night, but it's a choice I shouldn't have made. But at the time - there was just no way I wasn't going to play in that game. That's just the way I was.

I include this story so you can see that I was a young man with really no idea what I was ultimately going to do with my life. I had a high school diploma that I didn't really earn, I wasn't athletic enough to make a career out of sports (especially now with a bad right leg), and I didn't have any connections or prospects in the business world that could help me.

I knew this much – I wasn't going to go to college or university. I had to get a job. And so my working life began.

CHAPTER 3

WORKING LIFE

One thing I could do was talk. Make that I could bullshit! People who know me well won't be surprised to hear that!

My first real job was at Athlete's World in Yorkdale. It was the first of I guess five or six jobs I held from the time I was 18 until my 30s. All of them were in sales. I was good at sales. I had a real knack for it.

I knew how to talk to people and I knew how to sell. What I didn't know was the art of patience, as I got either tired or bored of jobs and wound up quitting so I could move on to the next opportunity. If I had just had the discipline to stick with one of these jobs for a while, I might have done some good things in the long term. But I just didn't have the patience.

I moved out of my parents' place and eventually I rented a room from a friend. I was basically just drifting through life in my early 20s, going from one job to another.

Some of the jobs were good, some not so good. I remember one job in particular I had – cold call selling for the Factory Blind Shop. Wow was that one tough!

It was a lot of cold calling. It was lots of rejection. I had more doors slammed in my face, more people telling me to f@&* off, than I ever imagined possible. People who have done this kind of work know what I'm talking about. You experience the worst in humanity at times, and you are subjected to true rejection and rejection after rejection. I really wonder sometimes if all that rejection I experienced in tough sales jobs like some of the ones I had back then led to the self-esteem issues I developed later on. It could very well be. All I know is the dejection I experienced made me feel as bad about myself as I did when I had my literacy problems in school.

Needless to say, the Factory Blind Shop gig was one that didn't last very long.

The highlight of this time period for me was definitely meeting my wife Cheryl. She ran a swim school at the time that I met her, and she was without doubt the best thing that had happened to me up until that point in my life. We were married on June 19, 1983. I was 23 and she was 21. It was great for my self-esteem to have a wife like her at the time let me tell you…and I sure needed that boost.

But now I was a married man with responsibilities, and before too long we discovered that our first child would soon be on the way. The kinds of jobs I had up until this point just weren't going to cut it anymore.

Cheryl had a good gig, but I felt the pressure to come up with a job that could make me a true breadwinner, someone who could properly look after his family.

I saw an ad for one that I knew would be a perfect fit. It was with Swiss Herbal Remedies, working as a salesperson reporting to their head office in Markham. The starting pay was $35,000 a year. I was making $15-17,000 at the time. It was too good to be true!

I polished up my resume and went in for an interview. I had made up my mind that I was not leaving that office until I got that job.

Well I got that job. But I got it by being a total liar and it wound up costing me dearly further down the road.

◘ ◘ ◘

Like I said, I can bullshit. I can talk to people. I know how to sell. But the greatest bullshit job and sales job I ever did was the number I pulled on this fine company in order to get that job.

I polished up my resume alright. I polished it up with bullshit. It was full of lies. Luckily for me, companies could not check out frauds back in those days the way they can now, or I would have been discovered for sure before I had even started working for them.

I wowed them in the interview with my passion, my commitment, my salesmanship…and my bullshit. I told them that I was the guy they needed, and they believed me. I was hired to cover the territory between Thunder Bay and Toronto, a huge area.

I need the job and I got the job…but it almost killed me.

There was no question that I was qualified to sell for Swiss Herbal Remedies or anybody else. I was qualified to sell anything with my mouth. What I wasn't qualified for were the technical requirements that came with the job. I knew nothing about the industry or how it worked.

But I fooled them into thinking I did, they hired me and off I went. I was travelling an awful lot, on the road all the time, desperately trying to make a living and not be discovered for the fraud that I really was.

I'd be on the road - one minute thinking to myself 'Rosey you are an incredible person who can do anything' after I made a big sale – to thinking 'Rosey you are a worthless piece of garbage' after I failed on a sale or had an especially rough day. I was on an emotional roller coaster all the time, always with the underlining fear that I would be discovered and fired for the fact that I had no idea what I was talking about. I was a total wreck.

It was bad enough pressure to be under when I only had a wife to look after. Then our baby came along…a wonderful occasion but it brought even more stress.

On October 15, 1984, our daughter Stephanie was born. I remember we were having Chinese food that night when Cheryl realized the baby was on its way.

It was a long labor…but not as long as the nurse who was caring for Cheryl thought it was going to be. That nurse told me it was going to be at least 15 hours before she gave birth. She said that I should just go home and wait. After she had delivered that news and left the room, Cheryl went into the bathroom and collapsed. The baby was on the way right then and there!

She wound up having the baby very soon after…I wanted to knock that nurse out! Thank God Cheryl was okay and the baby arrived safely, thanks to the help of the staff and the interns who were there.

At first I was told it was a boy. Then I was told it was a girl after the intern checked twice! But it was a healthy child, and I was so relieved and delighted that our baby and Cheryl were both safe and well.

Then it really hit me. 'Oh my God' I thought. 'I'm 24 years old and I have a baby.'

I was also working in a job that we really needed me to have and do well in, and I was totally bullshitting every moment I was there. But I couldn't afford to lose that job now, especially with Stephanie in the world.

After a short period of celebration, it was back on the road for me and back to my lies. What would happen to me if I was ever discovered? And what would happen to my family?

We were about to find out.

◘ ◘ ◘

Every day I worked in that job I lived in terror of being found out. I felt like a total fraud because that's what I really was. When it came to the products, I had no idea what I was talking about.

I had lied on my resume to get the job, I had no practical experience with, or knowledge about, the products I was selling, but I carried on the best I could. I needed the money.

Since I was on the road a lot, I had time to sit and think in the car. All I could think about was getting caught and losing the job. Then what would we do? I had a baby at home that I needed to provide for, so I put those thoughts aside and I kept this charade up for as long as I could.

It was excruciating for me. I'd be on a sales call and get questions about a certain product from a customer and I would have no idea how to answer it. I'd excuse myself for a few minutes, rush out to my car and call the chemist to get enough information to keep fooling them; I was fooling both the customers and my bosses at the same time.

I knew this couldn't last long and it didn't. Every day it went through my mind that I was going to get caught, get exposed, and after fooling everyone for close to a year sure enough one day it happened.

I was in a sales meeting with nowhere to go. The talk came around to me and it was obvious that I couldn't hack it technically to work in a position like this. I was totally out of my league and I got exposed right in front of many of my colleagues. I was sunk.

They let me go from the job. It devastated me. I lost the company car I had, the salary, all the benefits, and I was left with no car and no income. We were forced to move in with Cheryl's parents so we could continue to care for Stephanie.

I felt like a real failure. I felt like a total loser. It was right around this time that I really started using narcotics and alcohol on a serious basis. I felt my life was going nowhere and I turned to drugs and booze to help get me through it.

I was using drugs and drinking a lot. That only made things worse of course, but I didn't really care back then. A bad habit was starting to turn into a serious one.

For the next two years I must have had seven jobs, going from one to the other because I either quit or was fired. It was a miserable time all around.

Still we somehow managed, even with more mouths coming to feed. Sammy was born on April 13, 1986 and Nikki came along on May 22, 1988. They were blessings to us – then and now – but they did add to our load.

There was no job that I could hold for any decent length of time, and I began taking narcotics like they were skittles. I also began having serious issues with my leg again, and my answer to that was to take pain killers and drink too much to mask the pain, when the pain killers no longer did the trick.

It was a time in my life I am truly ashamed of. I was a terrible husband and a terrible father and I knew it. This pattern of behavior continued for the next several years. It felt like I was on a merry-go-round – I was never stopping but I was never getting anywhere, I was just going around in circles.

Sometime in 1993 – I don't remember exactly when – my wife found a bag of pills that I had hidden in the washroom, narcotics that I had been using to mask my pain, both the physical and the mental pain, that I was experiencing.

That was the end of fooling her once she discovered them. The irony of ironies was that her father was Chief Investigator for the Bureau of Dangerous Drugs. She was furious with me, and for good reason. Not only was I destroying my life, just imagine the shame she would have had to endure with her own family if they discovered I was using illegal substances. That would have been a very bad look for such a respected family in the community.

For the first time in my life, I went into rehab. I voluntarily admitted myself to Harmony House in Kirkland Lake for a period of 90 days to clean myself up. I knew I had to do it, to save myself and my marriage. I really had nothing to lose at that point, so I sought some professional help for my problems.

As it turned out, however, going to rehab only made my problems worse.

CHAPTER 4

REHAB WOES

Going into rehab is supposed to make you better. That is what I was told and that was what got me to go there voluntarily. But I wound up leaving there in worse shape than I was when I went in.

I had only been there a few days when one of the workers at the place offered to sell me narcotics! I don't know if that's the way it was for anybody else who was in rehab, but in my case…well let's just say I could get whatever I wanted in there without getting into the details. It was a total joke.

Checking into rehab was supposed to help me! But for the entire time there I was able to continue using drugs while I went through the motions of being rehabbed. I felt so much shame about what was happening inside there, but that didn't stop me from breaking the rules with the help of one of the workers. Honestly, I left there worse off than I was before I went in.

When I was released our problems continued. No surprise there. Cheryl finally had enough of me and my act in early 1994, and we split up.

I couldn't blame her, I really couldn't. But I still loved her and loved my kids. I really desperately wanted to be a good husband and father to them, but I couldn't hold a steady job and was still using narcotics and drinking too much to mask the pain I was feeling inside and outside. I felt deep down that I didn't deserve to have a good family life.

But after six months apart, Cheryl gave me what would be the first of a thousand second chances. We got back together. I'll never know why she kept believing that things would change, but she did. I was so grateful to her for that. She still had her career and she had kept our family together without me, yet still she gave me another chance by allowing us to reconcile.

Unfortunately nothing really changed, however. I did at least manage to hold on to a job for a bit, working for Squirrel Vending, a vending machine company, from 1994 to 1997. (Their slogan was "Nuts to you" which I loved!). I'd drive to the locations and service them and it was a decent job for a while, but it was nothing special. At least we were getting by, thanks to the steady employment.

My life plodded along. My disastrous stint in rehab hadn't helped, but I was managing to get up and go to work every day at least. And I still had some sports in my life, which helped keep me from going off the rails completely.

My love of sports had never left me. I was still playing some men's league hockey when I could and hanging out at The Rinks a lot whenever possible, just so I could stay in that environment. I always loved being in an arena and always felt at home there, so I played whenever the chance came around.

Being around the arena would lead to something important that happened to me early on in 1997. It didn't seem like a huge deal at the time, but it turned out to be a life changing moment when I look back on it now. It also inadvertently led to an obsession I got that would dominate my life for the next several years.

I was about to get a chance to coach some hockey for the first time - and I was about to meet a young man that I wound up spending more time with and attention on than I did with my own family.

My obsession with a young man named Max Birbraer would change my life...and his.

CHAPTER 5

MEETING MAX

Morrie Frydberg was a friend of mine who was connected to the Under-18 Israeli National hockey team. The team was slated to play at the Under-18 world championships in Belgrade, Yugoslavia and they were always looking for help as it was an extremely difficult task for Israel to ice a team.

Belgrade also wasn't a very safe place to be back in those days, especially if you were Jewish, and there were seven Canadian-born players who were going to be on the team. As a result of that, Morrie really felt that there should be a Canadian on the coaching staff to help look after the Canadian contingent.

As a result there was an opening for an Assistant Coach. There wasn't a lot happening in my life at that time, so when Morrie approached me about possibly helping out, I was really excited about the opportunity. It was in hockey, it would involve travelling to Yugoslavia for the world championships, and it seemed like a really cool thing to do. It sure beat any of the other things I had done in the past decade.

Trouble was it was a volunteer position. Taking time away from a job, that while not very engaging at least paid me, to volunteer to coach hockey, wasn't something I should have been doing at this particular time. However I sold it to Cheryl as it being a great opportunity for me that would lead to something bigger down the road.

I convinced her and my friends that this was going to be something fantastic for me. I agreed to go and serve as a volunteer assistant coach.

As it turned out, it was a great opportunity but for a completely different reason; that is where I first met Max Birbraer, a 16-year-old hockey player from Kazakhstan. He had played with Nik Antropov, who had made it to the National Hockey League with the Toronto Maple Leafs, and he was to become the focus of my life for basically the next few years.

I wound be concentrating more on Max's development than I did on our own team on that trip to Belgrade.

I was among eight Canadians who were involved with the Israeli team, which was led by the President Michael Budd. We arrived in Yugoslavia and started preparing for the event, and that's when I first laid eyes on Max.

From the time I first saw Max play in January, 1997 and heard his story, it didn't matter what our team did, the only thing that mattered was that I had to help this kid get an opportunity to do what Nik Antropov did, and that was play in the NHL.

We hit it off immediately after I was introduced to him. I watched him score two brilliant goals in a game against Yugoslavia, and I realized right away this kid had the potential to play pro hockey if he got some direction and some help. I became determined to be the person who would help him do that.

Max spoke Russian and Hebrew and I spoke only English, but we still found a way to communicate. He clearly needed some help in navigating his path so he could take advantage of his tremendous abilities. He needed a lot of help with a lot of things; for instance, he was wearing size 11 skates and he should have been in size 8, but it was the only pair he could get.

I had taken the volunteer coaching job to help the Israeli team with the hope it might lead to something else in hockey down the road. However the end result from that decision was that I wound up becoming Max's mentor and guardian for many years as he attempted to break away from Kazakhstan and become a player in the NHL in North America.

I'm going to talk a lot about Max shortly, but I should say something about another thing I got from my experience with the Israeli team. I saw firsthand how horrible anti-Semitism can be.

The hatred directed towards the Israeli team wherever it went in Belgrade was palatable. We had to be escorted off the ice after some games, with some fans threatening us. It was truly an eye-opening experience to experience how deep some people's hatred runs.

We visited a memorial to Holocaust survivors while we were there. During that visit a young kid, no more than 10 or 11 years old, spit in my face and called me "a fucking Jew" because I was wearing an Israeli track suit issued by the team.

You can imagine how angry and appalled I was. But that turned out to be a teaching moment for me. I knew it wouldn't do any good to be angry, or to lash out, at a small kid. Racism was mired in him obviously; it came from his background. A child like that doesn't hate like that unless the hate is instilled in him. I realized he just didn't know any different, which made me more sad than angry. That moment has stayed with me since and helped me deal with other anti-semantic behavior I've witnessed over the years.

The experience with the Israeli Under-18 team was a valuable one for me in many ways. I got to help coach a group of fine young men; I got to proudly wear the Israeli colors, and learned a lot about myself and my being Jewish in the process. But all of that pales in comparison to meeting Max and what that meeting led to for me in the next few years.

To be honest, Max Birbraer wound up becoming more important to me than my own family.

◙ ◙ ◙

I admit this fully right here and now as I promised you I was going to be totally honest in this book – it was awful of me to ignore my own family and turn all of my attention onto Max, even though he clearly needed help from someone.

Here is my poor wife, taking care of our house and our three kids, and she's paying for everything. And what am I doing? I'm doing everything I can to make sure Max gets to the NHL and make his dreams of playing there come to life. And to make matters worse, I would have never met Max unless I had taken a volunteer coaching job.

Max wound up living with our family from 1997 to 1999 as he came to North America to chase his hockey dream. He played for the Newmarket Hurricanes and immediately showed that he was indeed a bona-fide prospect. However Cheryl now has another mouth to feed as I spend all of my time trying to open as many doors as I could for Max.

It was not a great time for me personally as I played this role of mentor/guardian/quasi-agent for Max. I still had an insane drug habit that I couldn't shake, and I couldn't hold on to a decent paying job for very long. But I had Max to look after and that in my mind gave my life some sort of meaning.

I admit that I was a terrible burden to my own family, and that they needed the kind of support that I was trying to give to Max. They should have been my top priority. But deep down I wanted Max to succeed so badly, and I felt that if I could help him, it might lead to something bigger for me in hockey down the road as well. If I could be remembered as the guy who brought a future superstar into the NHL, it might create a role for me as an agent, scout or whatever. I fully admit that was part of my thinking.

I should mention that I received a lot of help with Max from my friend Joe Arfin. He also saw the potential that Max had and he really helped me out, especially taking care of Max when I couldn't. He stepped up and played a huge role in helping me with Max's success, especially after I started really having some serious health issues.

My health was getting worse during these years, especially my leg, and that wasn't helping matters any. My leg had given way when I was in Frankfurt in April 1997, and in July of that year I had a knee replacement. I picked up a wicked infection after that surgery. Combined with my drug and alcohol abuse, I was in bad shape physically and mentally at a time where I needed to be as sharp as possible.

But I put my health at extreme risk and pressed on, not for my family, but because I was looking after Max. And at the start, things were looking pretty good for him after I managed to get him to North America.

He was drafted by the New Jersey Devils with the 62nd overall pick in the 2000 NHL Draft, and was sent to the Albany River Rats, the Devils' American Hockey League team, to continue his development.

I would drive everywhere to see him play in all of his games. I even followed him to Albany and moved in with him for a time to keep tabs on him. Meanwhile my wife is holding the fort at home while I'm out risking my health and sanity over Max's career. What the hell was I doing here?

I even took legal guardianship of him, and eventually I was introduced to Brad Robbins of KSR Sports, the firm run by Gord Kirke and Gord Stellick. I eventually gave Max to Brad so he could manage him properly, and I was promised that if the kid ever signed a big contract I would be looked after.

I'll have more about Max later in this book, as he remained a big part of my life and still is actually, even to this day. I loved the kid and only wanted what was best for him, I really did. But my preoccupation with helping him to succeed turned me into a wreck, both physically and mentally, and it came at the expense of my own family.

My leg was killing me back then too. I was in so much pain. From 1997 to 1999, when I was handling Max, I must have had 20 procedures of some kind to try and make it better, while at the same time self-medicating myself with drugs and alcohol. During those years if I wasn't in the hospital dealing with my leg issues, I was with Max…either on the road, or in Albany. Meanwhile my wife soldiered on with my own family while I was rarely home.

Honestly, I don't know how I survived. But somehow I did.

My leg, however, did not.

CHAPTER 6

LOSING LIMB

Everything happens for a reason, or so they say. As you will find out in later chapters of this book, there was even an important reason that I lost my leg.

It was impossible to see that reason for losing a limb when it happened to me, however.

I knew I was in bad shape physically overall during this time period. My leg had been an issue for many years as you've already read, but I still kept living this reckless lifestyle of mine.

I was all over the place chasing Max. I was abusing my body with drugs and alcohol. My knee replacement in 1997 resulted in serious infections that never really cleared up. I was basically a ticking time bomb.

In June of 1999, I travelled to Israel to see a doctor I knew there about my leg. I had a connection there with some medical people and I felt that I could get some treatment or a proper diagnosis of what exactly was wrong with my leg from them.

I wasn't feeling well at all. I was in constant pain so on June 8, I went to Israel to see that doctor in hopes that he could help me.

The news I was given was grim. Very grim.

"You've got a serious infection and if you don't get to a hospital, you are going to die, this is going to kill you," I was told. I was just stunned. Despite knowing deep down that something was seriously wrong with my leg, I had no idea it was this serious. I had made this trip to get cured, not to be told I was on the verge of dying.

That was June 8, 1999. The next day, June 9, doctors amputated my right leg at mid-thigh in order to stave off the deadly infection that was spreading and save my life. I was told after the amputation if I had waited any longer, I might not have made it.

It was that fast. Just like that, I had become an amputee. Just like that, I was facing an enormous new challenge…living life with just one leg.

My foolish lifestyle decisions had finally caught up with me.

⊡ ⊡ ⊡

I wound up spending 14 days in Israel as a result of the amputation, four of them confined in the hospital. To say I was totally stunned and totally discouraged at that point would be an understatement.

A completely different way of living was now being forced upon me. I would have to find a way to live with one limb and make all of the adjustments that would be necessary in order to do that.

I was 39 years old. I had a wife and three kids. I had no real career prospects. And I was down to one leg.

Shortly after the surgery I came back home to Canada to begin my rehabilitation. I was eventually fitted with a prosthetic and went through the process of learning to properly walk with one.

My rehab started at Hillcrest, where I was surrounded by mostly old people. It was a depressing, difficult time as I tried to adjust to a new life missing a limb, but deep down I guess I also realized that I could have very easily died. Losing a limb is bad, but death is far worse. I somehow found the courage to learn to live with this disability and just be happy that it hadn't killed me.

There was a lot wrong in my life at this point, but I was still alive. That was the only way to look at it, I had determined in my own mind. The shock of having had the amputation had worn off but the shock of almost having died had not, which was a good thing for me. I tried to look at it not as losing a limb, but as winning a second chance at living. I really came frighteningly close to dying, so despite the massive loss I found comfort in just being here I suppose.

I knew one thing for sure; I had to stay active or I would go insane. I had to find something to keep me busy and to keep my mind and my body active.

Fortunately I discovered a place called Variety Village, where I went to further my rehab.

Thank God for Variety Village. It literally saved my life and helped send it in a direction I would never have dreamed of.

❏ ❏ ❏

I cannot say enough good things about Variety Village on Danforth Avenue in Scarborough, Ontario and the people who make the existence of such a terrific facility possible.

Variety Village is operated by the Variety Club of Ontario and it's a place where healing happens. It certainly did happen there for me, as it allowed me to continue my rehab while being treated with respect. I needed to get into shape and concentrate on what I could do after the amputation, instead of what I couldn't do. It was the perfect place for me to do that.

I knew I had to stay busy after losing my leg, especially doing something physical. If I let my thoughts about the amputation run wild, the reality of what had happened would take over and I'd be depressed. I was almost euphoric about getting a second chance at life, but that would soon wear off if I didn't look for the positives from this blow I had been dealt.

So I went there and started working out and participating in whatever sports I could. I threw myself into every program they offered and into my rehab.

It was a real blessing. The place is world class and I was able to keep moving in a positive environment. And one of the best things about it was the great people who also went there for the same reasons that brought me.

One of them was Shane Smith. He was a triple amputee, having lost one arm and both of his legs. What a terrific man he is, and what an inspiration he was coming into my life just when I needed it. If he wasn't going to be stopped by what happened to him I sure wasn't going to be either.

Every one of us needs people we can look up to, especially in difficult times. Shane was that to me and so much more.

Shane became like a son to me as I got to know him. I owe him a lot just for helping me to get over losing my leg, but the thing I owe him for the most was something else he did for me.

Shane introduced me to something called sledge hockey. He changed my life with that introduction.

CHAPTER 7

SLEDGE HOCKEY

Like most people I suppose, I had no idea what sledge hockey was or what was involved in playing it. All I knew was that I wanted to find a sport that I could still enjoy, since clearly my beer league hockey playing days were over with one leg left.

Shane was involved with the Markham Islanders, a sledge hockey team. He opened my eyes to what this sport was all about.

It was still hockey, he explained to me. You can still play hockey on a sledge. Shane sold me on the idea of giving the sport a try and I got hooked on it fast.

I developed a real passion for it…mostly at first just because it was fun! And it was still hockey. I started playing this great sport because of Shane and for that I'll always be thankful to him.

Shane was a godsend for me in so many ways. He was so inspiring. And as a result of his inspiration, I also started modeling his actions by trying to help others in their struggles after losing a limb.

I remember one time I agreed to do a talk to some kids at Sick Kids Hospital. On the way to the talk, I decided that I would shave my head (and I had some pretty good looking hair back then!) just to show my support for the kids who were losing their hair while undergoing chemo. I'll never forget seeing a 10-year-old kid that day who had lost his hair, and the smile on his face when I told him I had lost my hair too!

That really marked the start of me trying to help others with my public speaking skills. If it weren't for Shane, I might not have gone down that road later in my life as well. As you'll read later on in this book, motivational speaking became a lucrative sideline for me. Like I said, I owe Shane a lot.

Once I had decided that I was going to try sledge hockey, I embraced it fully. With everything I have ever done in my life, I've always felt you can never be concerned about what people think, you just have to go out there and do it. Sledge hockey looks a bit odd when you first see it and some people might chuckle at it – I couldn't have cared less. I quickly discovered it took a lot of skill to stay on the sledge and play the game.

I got accustomed to the sledge relatively quickly and after some extra practice, learned to get around the ice pretty well on it. Shane then surprised me by asking me if I would consider being a goaltender.

A goaltender? Where did that come from?! I had never been a goalie in my life. I'd played forward in hockey and I was a catcher in baseball, but being a goaltender was something I had never tried. But Shane asked me if I would because his team needed one, and since this was a new sport for me, I said sure, I'd give it a whirl.

My first game in goal will go down in the history books as a loss. 1-0 was the final score. But we were out-shot 53-3 – that's right, 53-3, I'll never forget that! I had allowed just one goal despite having to face all those shots. No wonder they wanted me to play in goal they were probably expecting me to get hammered!

I caught on to the position pretty quickly obviously. And the exhilaration I felt as a result of being successful at something in sports did my mental health a lot of good.

My performance didn't go unnoticed in sledge hockey circles. Shane in particular was really impressed, and he informed me that Team Canada was looking for another goalie and that I should try out for the team.

Whoa! Wait a minute – there's a Team Canada sledge hockey team?

Like I said, I was pretty new to the sport. I had no idea. But what national team would even consider letting me try out for them?

I was excited by the thought and of course I was going to take advantage of that opportunity. However I knew that I would have to get really serious about this sport and train my ass off before I did that. But with just one game under my belt I was already on my way to maybe getting a chance to audition for Team Canada…it was a pretty incredible development now that I look back on it.

Here's something else about that day of my first game that I'll never forget.

I came home after playing and my daughter Stephanie greets me by asking, "How was sledge hockey, Dad?"

"Pretty good," I told her. "Looks like I am going to try out for Team Canada."

She looked at me and just laughed and shook her head. She thought I was nuts. I had only played one game, but now I had a national team tryout?!

We both had no idea back then what was in store for me with Team Canada.

CHAPTER 8

TEAM CANADA

Okay. So my sledge hockey career is obviously off to a roaring start, but there was no way I was just going to show up to Team Canada and take their offer of a tryout just hoping for the best. I went to work first.

And when I say I went to work, I mean I really went to work!

I didn't just want to get a tryout for Team Canada; I wanted to MAKE the team. And despite obviously being a "natural" in goal, and there clearly being a need for another goalie (who wants to play goal in sledge hockey after all, all the fun is playing up front!), I realized I needed to be the best I could be before showing them what I could do for them in goal.

I met Jamie McGuire who was a goalie coach and convinced him to work with me. And off to work I went, training every chance I could get, with Jamie guiding me every step of the way.

And I didn't just train with other sledge hockey players. I actually wound up training with some of the best stand up hockey players in the world, which was a tremendous advantage for me.

My reasoning for this was simple. I had a lot of respect for the sledge hockey players, they were terrific athletes. But I felt that if I could learn to stop some truly great shooters who were standing in front of my sledge, it would make me that much better in sledge hockey competitions. It only made sense. My training would be harder than the actual games would be, and this attitude and plan I brought was the biggest reason that when I did try out for Team Canada, I made the team.

McGuire was tough on me boy. One of the first shots he took on me was absolute cannon that hit me right in the face. I guess he wanted to see what I was made of right away and when I didn't back down, we really got to work.

I trained with him for six months, and thanks to his connections, I got to handle shots from some NHL players who were looking to keep sharp in the off-season. Players like NHL regulars Kyle Quincey and Shane Corson were shooting on me. It was frankly terrifying at first! But once I got used to handling the quality of their shots, everything else I faced became much easier to handle.

How many other sledge hockey goalies were getting that kind of big-time practice? Easy answer to that one – none of them were, just me. I had a real advantage when it came time to show what I could do, and that time came when I got a chance to try out for Team Canada in May of 2001.

◘ ◘ ◘

When it came time for the tryouts I was ready to go. I had faced big league shooters and held my own, so my confidence was sky high as I went to the tryouts in Ottawa.

Sledge hockey wasn't receiving any funding back then. None. So when I drove to Ottawa for my tryout, I had to cover all my expenses and pay $50 to boot just for the privilege of trying out for a national team. But that didn't stop me as I really believed I would make the team after all the work I had put in.

Dean Delaurier was the President of Canadian Sled Hockey at that time. Here I was, I had just turned 41 years old, and I was sitting at a table with him and two other guys as I got ready for the tryouts. I'm sure they were laughing at this old fart who was trying out and happy to take my 50 bucks. I on the other hand was just happy to have the opportunity.

They had no idea who I was before that tryout. They also had no idea of all of the work I had put in back at Variety Village to make all of this possible. I went in there thinking I had 48 hours to impress these guys and that's exactly what I set out to do.

They sure knew who I was at the end of the tryout. I made the team. I was going to get to wear the Team Canada colors.

From that moment on, being the best sledge hockey goalie I could be became my life's mission. I had found my passion and I was going to make the best of it.

I set three goals for myself before I even stepped on the ice for the first time wearing the Team Canada colors.

Goal one was to make the team. Goal two was that by 2006 (five years from then), I was going to be the best sledge hockey goalie in the world. Goal three was that by the time I retired, I was going to be in the Hockey Hall of Fame in some capacity (I vowed to do something so good on the ice that I would get mentioned in the Hall and it would leave a lasting impact).

Cocky? Yes I guess I was. But my confidence came as a result of the work that I had done to prepare for this. Losing my leg turned out to be the catalyst in giving me the greatest opportunity of my life – I was going to play for Team Canada and make my name in a sport that was still growing.

From the moment I had the amputation, I believed deep down that there had to be a reason for this to have happened. Here it was. Becoming disabled had allowed me the opportunity to also become a disabled athlete at the national level.

I wound up having a terrific run for about a decade as one of the best sledge hockey goalies in the world and I'm very proud of it. But as good a player as I was, I was an even bigger help to Team Canada and the sport off the ice with another great weapon I had.

My mouth.

CHAPTER 9

PR MAN

So I am on the team. I am the 41-year-old back-up goalie on Team Canada's sledge hockey team to the starter, Pierre Pichette.

I was fine with that (although he wasn't which I'll get into later). But as nice sounding as it was to be called a national athlete, it was also expensive. Money was something I didn't have a lot of.

Not only was there no money in playing sledge hockey in 1999, you had to PAY to play sledge hockey. Every player had to come up with $2,500 to cover the costs of playing in major tournaments, and the sport was desperate to get government and corporate funding to help cover those costs.

This wasn't the NHL. This hockey party was BYOC – bring your own cash.

You've read this far into the book so you know my sales background by now. And you have probably figured out already that I can talk. So I put both of those skills to good use in trying to help change the financial position our sport was in even before playing.

We had to pay to play, so I went out pitching the sport to everyone I knew, and everyone I didn't know, looking to get our team properly funded. I went to news outlets everywhere pleading our case, and I wasn't shy about it either.

I had only recently joined the team, so you might be wondering why I was the guy doing all of this. Simple reason – I had a big mouth and was willing to advocate for people with disabilities. Other veteran players weren't as outgoing as I was. In my early years with the team I spent more time making funding pitches than I did playing, but I was happy to help out the cause anyway I could.

Throughout my career it was promote, promote, promote as much as it was play, play, play…and that was OK by me. I relished the role of being the sport's go-to promoter right from the start.

Here's a side story here for minute about a memorable day when I was out promoting.

On September 5, 2001, The Hockey News asked me to do a photo shoot with them to help promote the sport. I was delighted to do it and went to Thornhill, just outside Toronto, for the photo session on September 11.

I'll never forget that day, as we all won't. While I was doing the photo shoot in the morning, the 9/11 attacks were underway in New York. It was a terrifying day for all of us, but I had no idea of the enormity of what had happened until we were finished with our picture taking session.

Max was with the New Jersey Devils at the time and they were actually planning to visit the World Trade Center that very day. The plan was for them to get their medicals done for the start of the season at the excellent facilities they had there, and they were on their way to the Towers that morning. That visit never happened of course, and it just goes to show how fragile life can be. The first phone call I made after I found out what had happened was to Max, to make sure he was OK.

They were fine, as the planes hit the towers long before they were scheduled to arrive. I was okay too as I wasn't near the site, but thousands of others lost their lives that day and hundreds of thousands of their loved ones' lives were permanently changed as a result.

You never know what can happen friends. Your life can turn on a dime. I sure knew that first hand.

◘ ◘ ◘

So as the new millennium begins and the new decade moves long, I'm the back-up goalie/promoter for Team Canada's sledge hockey team.

Meanwhile my wife is holding down the family court and Max is slowly making his way in pro hockey. I'm still drinking too much, using narcotics and not really earning a living, but I'm hopeful all this hockey related work is going to pay off financially at some point (sound familiar?).

As the back-up goalie I'm not playing much at all, but I had come so far in the sport so quickly I wasn't complaining. I was wearing a Team Canada jersey, I was travelling to tournaments all over the place and I was willing to pay my dues and wait for my chance to one day be the number one goalie.

As much as I was enjoying it, it wasn't easy let me tell you. It might have been, but Pierre Pichette made it tougher for me than it should have been. I guess he felt threatened by me and resented the fact that I had made my way onto the team so quickly. I think he also resented the fact that I was doing all the talking to try and raise funds for the team and getting a lot of publicity. I wasn't playing much, but most people saw me as the spokesman for sledge hockey because I did so much talking in public about it.

For whatever the reason, Pierre and I did not get along and that was unfortunate. We were even roommates on one of our trips and he barely spoke to me, he just ignored me the whole time. That was bad enough, but it was made even worse by the fact that Pierre was extremely popular with his teammates, so some of his animosity towards me spread to other players as well. Our relationship just made things more difficult for both of us.

In October, 2001 we went to Norway and Sweden for tournaments in preparation for the upcoming 2002 Winter Olympics and Paralympics. Those Games were nearly cancelled by the 9/11 attacks, but fortunately they weren't. These warm-up events that we had were important as a result.

I mostly sat and watched, but whenever I got my chance I ran with it. In the fourth game of the tournament in Norway I got a rare start. Well I stood on my head and I was great as we win the game 1-0.

I felt pretty damn good about my performance in that game. But it turned out to be a bad thing for me because I was probably too good, which was a threat to Pierre. And since he was so popular, some of the guys on the team didn't like the fact that I was a threat to him either.

He (and some others on the team too) thought I never put the proper amount of training into the sport to get on the team. Also the only training I had prior to joining the team was with former NHL players, which they might have seen as disrespectful towards sledge hockey players. I was a bit of an outcast I suppose, so that performance in Norway didn't get me any more playing time, likely more out of respect for Pierre.

There was nothing I could do about that and our coach at the time Pierre Schweda made it clear that he was going to stay with his guy. I was disappointed, but I could live with it because we were going to the Olympics.

Back-up goalie or not, I was going to be a Paralympic athlete. What a thrill!

CHAPTER 10

FIRST PARALYMPICS

It's March 11, 2002. We are in Salt Lake City for the opening ceremonies of the 2002 Winter Paralympics. Wow.

I am overcome by the spectacle of it all. A packed crowd greets us as we are marched into the stadium to begin the biggest sporting event in the world. I can't believe this is happening to me, especially at my age and so quickly.

My eyes are filled with tears at one point. Here I am, after all of what I have been through, and I am standing on the field in a stadium wearing a Team Canada track suit with thousands of fans looking at us. We were all celebrating the joy and excitement that only an Olympic Games can bring.

My teammate and roomie for the Games, Shawn Matheson, is right next to me.

"Rosey, are you all right?" Shawn asks me with genuine concern, seeing how red my eyes were.

I can only nod, I can't even find the words to speak. Yes I'm all right. I just can't get over the fact that less than three years removed from losing my leg, here I am walking out here in Team Canada colors in the opening ceremonies for the Olympic Games!

It's a moment I will cherish forever and certainly never forget. But all was not well with our team as the Games were about to begin, however.

❏ ❏ ❏

Whenever the sport is hockey, the expectations are that Canada is going to win. Men's team, woman's team, or sledge hockey team doesn't matter – you play for Canada. You are supposed to win. There is only one color of medal that is acceptable and we all know what color it is.

But I knew there was no way we were going to win the gold medal in those Olympic Games. I knew we were in serious trouble right from the start, to be honest about it. We had no structure to our team, and our players weren't buying in to what our coaching staff was trying to tell us.

Team United States on the other hand, coached by former NHL great Rick Middleton, was fully invested in what its coaching staff was telling them. They were a vastly superior team to us as a result and we weren't going to have a chance against them unless we got better in a hurry.

We didn't. The Olympic Games are no place to start trying to get better. You are supposed to peak as a team just in time for the Olympics if you expected to win, and we didn't.

The off-shoot of that was that I got to play however. But my chance only came after our number one goalie basically pulled the shoot on us.

We were playing the Americans early in the tournament and frankly it was an embarrassment. They totally dominated us right from the start of the game and roared into a 4-0 lead at the end of the first period. To make matters worse, we faced a 5-on-3 disadvantage to start the second period.

It was pretty much a hopeless cause. When you are at a two-man disadvantage in sledge hockey, the other team usually scores - that's just the way it is.

I watched all this from my seat on the bench of course, as usual. Our dressing room was not a happy place to say the least as we filed in for the intermission.

It was then that I got the news from the coaching staff.

"You're going in Rosey" I was told. Our number one goalie had an "injury" they said to me and I was going to start the second period.

What the hell?! I am going in now, with a two-man disadvantage and a 4-0 deficit after one period? Talk about a can't win situation to put a guy into!

My teammate Billy Bridges started firing a roll of tape at me to help me get warmed up while we were still in the room. I had five minutes to get ready for my debut in the Paralympics in front of thousands of fans, and in a hopeless game situation.

I never knew what the "injury" Pichette had or even if he really actually had one; I just knew that after being totally ignored as the back-up, I was being sent into the game at the toughest possible time. Or I guess I could say I was being sent into the lion's den.

Into the goal I go. My Olympics debut begins and 20 seconds into it, the Americans do what most sledge hockey teams do on a 5-on-3 – they score. One shot on me so far, one goal, and it is 5-0 for the USA.

Welcome to the Paralympics Paul Rosen!

It was a tough spot, but I made the best of it. In fact, I didn't allow another goal the rest of the way in an eventual 5-1 loss to the Americans. That loss demonstrated clearly that there was no way we were winning a gold medal in these Olympics.

I'm not particularly proud of what I did next, but here's what I did after that game ended - I staged a bit of a mutiny.

I was furious. Not just furious because of the circumstances I was thrown into, but furious with the entire way the team was being coached and handled. As I mentioned earlier, we had no structure whatsoever.

Since I was the spokesman for the team, I decided to do some talking right there in the dressing room. I called a players only meeting, without our coaches Pierre Schweda and Tom Goodings in the room, and really let off some steam about the way things were going. This was the biggest sporting event in the world, I shouted, and we were playing like losers. It just wasn't acceptable.

I over-stepped my bounds. I admit it. I was a passionate guy and I was trying to do my part to get us going, but I shouldn't have done it. And worse still, it didn't help the team one bit.

I was shut down in that meeting pretty fast. The veterans on the team took exception to the way I spoke, especially what I said in regards to Pichette, who was the room's favorite. The meeting accomplished nothing and needless to say, the rest of those Olympics weren't very much fun for me as a result.

I didn't see much more playing time at all (just a 3-3 tie against Estonia) as Pichette immediately recovered from his "injury" and didn't miss another minute. We wound up finishing a very disappointing fourth.

That first Olympics remains a highlight for me because of the opening ceremonies and just being there. But I was all about winning a gold medal and we didn't; we weren't even close, so I wasn't a happy camper at all by the end of those Games.

The Team Canada brass obviously weren't happy either, as Schweda was fired shortly after we got home and eventually replaced by Peter Hambly.

Despite finishing fourth, it was a strong start in sledge hockey for me personally as I'd accomplished a lot already. I was on Team Canada. I was getting a reputation as an important spokesperson for getting funding for athletes with disabilities. Max was finding his way in pro hockey. There was a reason to hope for better days despite not bringing a medal home from Salt Lake City.

In the meantime however, I had to get back to my wife and family and make a living. The sledge hockey was all well and good, but it didn't pay the bills.

I did manage to make a living for a while too…moving dead bodies.

CHAPTER 11

FUNERAL BUSINESS

I've already talked about the many jobs I had in my life up until this point that I really hated. I want to take some time now to talk about a job that I had around this time period that I truly loved.

I made a good living working with the dead.

While it was great that I had found a passion for sledge hockey and made it to the Olympics, it still didn't pay the bills. Thank God again for my wife, who basically carried the household for so many years and continued to do so for most of the time that we were married for. But on June 5, 2000, I found a job that I wound up keeping for six years and was a true pleasure to have.

I was a dead body "removal expert" for Benjamin's Park Memorial Chapel.

After I had recovered from my leg amputation and discovered the joys of sledge hockey, I still needed to work. When I first made Team Canada there was no funding for the players, so I was faced with a real problem. I had to get a job to help my wife with the bills and still find the time to put in to being the best sledge hockey player that I could be.

Enter Benjamin's.

I somehow managed to get hired with that terrific company and it turned out to be one of the best places I ever worked. It was at the funeral home, it paid $30,000 a year and it had full benefits. The manager was Greg Gates, one of the finest people I ever worked for.

I really needed the job and I wanted to demonstrate that right from the start. Benjamin's has its own people picking up the dead bodies to transport them to the morgue or to the home, they didn't use outside help for that part of their business like some funeral homes did. Their clients were all Jewish families, and that religion requires people to be picked up and buried within

24 hours, so that particular part of the funeral process was pretty important to them.

As you can imagine however, it isn't the most pleasant job in the world sometimes. It involves handling a corpse and getting it ready for the funeral. It isn't a job for the squeamish.

I jumped at the opportunity to do that part of the business, however. I wanted to show them that I was somebody who cared, who took the role very seriously, and would treat any dead body that I had to handle with dignity and respect.

The first body I had to look after gave me a sense of how difficult a task this could be at times. It was a man who was sitting in a chair after a heroin overdose. It gave me the chills at first, but I kept my composure and looked after him.

Over my six years there I saw tons of suicides (many which were not made public), some murders and some other really ghastly situations. I'd have nightmares about some of the corpses that I had to work with; it could be a really difficult thing to do.

When I told people about what I did, most of them were fascinated by it. I became known as the "grim reaper of goaltenders" among some of my teammates for instance. It could be morbid at times for sure, but I truly loved working with Benjamin's. I had great respect for the company and for my boss, and I loved being able to keep people's minds at ease, knowing that their loved ones would be well looked after and with dignity and respect.

To be honest, I didn't want to leave this job, unlike the many other jobs I'd had that I couldn't wait to get out of. My bosses were very generous to me in letting me set my own schedule due to my Team Canada obligations, which really helped me a great deal. However that didn't go over very well with a lot of guys that I worked with. I guess I could see their point, it was becoming a bit of an issue. I was getting time off that they couldn't get and there was no way that situation could be allowed to continue. There was no way I was prepared to give up playing for Team Canada for any job, and so I had to leave a few months before the Olympic Games in Torino, Italy in 2006.

Still, I had no regrets. I understood the situation and I left with no ill feelings at all to anyone, either my bosses or my co-workers. They were all great people.

I remain truly thankful to them for giving me that opportunity. For the first time in my life I had found some paying work that I truly enjoyed and in an environment where my work was respected as well. It just couldn't continue to work with my hockey commitments and growing speaking career.

My involvement at Benjamin's made me an expert at dealing with corpses and that would lead me to an experience that still in many ways haunts me to this day – I was the person who prepared my own mother for the funeral home when she passed away in 2016.

If that sounds morbid to you, well I guess it is. But my mother had wanted me to do that for her, she had told me that many times while I was working there, and I knew that was a final wish of hers.

There was a part of me that wanted to do it for her, but there was a bigger part of me that found the idea terrible. I was really torn about this, but at the personal request of my mother and with Benjamin's permission, I took care of her body at the end.

I knew I was fulfilling a wish of hers, but it's something that somebody else should have done. I had performed these duties many times on other people, but the emotional toll caring for my Mom on me was really too much for me to bear.

You read at the start of the book that I would later try to take my own life in 2019. You saw how I was especially careful to have a shower and change into clean clothes before I took all those pills, preparing myself before anybody found my body. I wanted to be as clean and decent as possible for when my body was discovered. It was heart wrenching for me to make those preparations on that terrible night.

Now you know why.

CHAPTER 12

TOP GOALIE

With the 2002 Olympics behind us, Team Canada had a lot of work to do. The team had been basically falling apart by the time Jeff Snyder took over as head coach the summer after the Olympics.

When a new coach comes in to any team, there's basically a feeling out session for a while and that's what we went through I suppose during that time period. We continued to train and play in some tournaments with the eye on the 2004 world championships, which would hopefully lead to some redemption for us from our fourth place Paralympics finish.

For me this time was all about trying to convince team management and my teammates that I was the answer to our problems in goal. I wanted that net to myself and I was confident that if I was playing every game, we'd be far better off as a team.

Pierre Pichette was gone by now off to retirement, so there was myself and Greg Westlake as the two remaining goalies. We both deserved to play but that wasn't good enough for me – I wanted the number one job and like I said, I never wanted to sit and watch somebody else play goal for Team Canada. If I wasn't playing, I wasn't happy.

Greg was a good goalie, but he could also play forward and play it extremely well. The best course of action therefore for me and for the team, in my mind, was for him to play up front.

I was convinced we'd be a better team that way, with me in goal and Greg out of the crease playing up front. This became an ongoing discussion for us for the next year or so, as I did everything to convince everybody associated with the team that I should be the only man in goal.

The 2004 world championships were in Sweden. We were still very much a work in progress as a team. Greg and I both played some in goal in that tournament, but it wasn't a great one for Team Canada by any stretch of the imagination.

In all my years of playing I was only pulled from a game once and it happened at the 2004 worlds. It was in the bronze medal game against Sweden when we were down 3-0. I'm sure you can easily imagine how I felt about being yanked.

We wound up losing that game anyway and finished fourth. Once again, no medal for a Canadian hockey team in international competition. It was extremely disappointing.

The next Paralympics were in 2006 in Torino, Italy, and that obviously became the focus for us after yet another tough defeat. We had to find a way to get better…and I had the answer of course. It was for Greg Westlake to move out of the net and Paul Rosen to move into the net full-time.

I was adamant that this was the right thing to do. I kept calling Jeff Snyder and bugging him to see it my way, and I kept putting the idea into Greg's head that he should play forward too (he was my roommate on the road for five years so I had a lot of time to try and convince him!). My reasoning was that our number one line would then be the best in the world, our number two line could also score and play defense and our number three line was our shut down line.

And of course, Paul Rosen could then play every single game in goal with no worries. That was really my main motivation. My teammates saw through my plans and at times, it created some tensions in the dressing room.

My roommate in Salt Lake City Shawn Matheson and I got along great, but even we argued about the back-up goalie situation. It became a major issue with me and affected the way I interacted with my Team Canada coach and teammates.

Looking back on this "goalie controversy" now, I can see why a lot of people hated my guts. I fully admit I was a bit of an asshole. I didn't care about making friends, I just wanted to win. I had a big ego, I knew I was good, and I had to feed that ego.

I was really driven to succeed, to the point that I was a real ass about it. It was the way I was wired and although I am not proud about the way I acted, it was that intense drive to win that made me the goalie that I was. Still, it wasn't an easy time for us as a team and I certainly wasn't an easy guy to be around because of my attitude.

It would take a while for everybody to come around to my way of thinking on this issue, but they eventually did. I'd get my wish and be the number one goalie and Greg would turn out to be a tremendous forward for us. However it took a lot of convincing on my part over the next two years for it to finally happen.

2004-2005 was one of the craziest times of my life for that reason and several others. I was going a million miles a minute. Between training for and playing in tournaments, along with promoting the team at every opportunity, I was probably on the road about 200 days a year over that two year period leading up to the Torino Games. That's a lot of time to be spending on something that doesn't pay your bills.

We still had no funding. We were still basically paying to play. It was still a joke frankly, and something had to be done about it. It would turn out that I was going to be the person who did something.

CHAPTER 13

COACHING CANADA

Before I continue my story about playing for Team Canada and the battle that was ahead to get us some funding, I want to take a moment to talk about my involvement with the Canadian Amputee Hockey Team.

As I was starting my career as a goalie in sled hockey, I was also looking for other ways I could to be a part of athletics. Finding a sport I could play was a Godsend, but thanks to the Canadian Amputee hockey team, I was also able to get involved in coaching.

After losing my leg in 1999, I tried to skate but there was no way I could. So sled hockey became my playing fix and as it would turn out, the Canadian Amputee hockey team would provide me with an opportunity to coach.

These guys were incredible athletes and it was an honor to coach them. Amputee hockey is not a Paralympic sport, but the players are incredible. They are all amputees who have found a way to still play a sport they love at a very high level, and it was just such a tremendous experience to be able to coach them.

I went to check the sport out in 2000 and I was blown away by the players' passion for the game and the skill they were able to demonstrate on the ice. When they approached me to coach the team, it was a true honor and although my life was all over the place during this timeframe (as you've just read), I couldn't say no.

We had some terrific success as well, winning gold medals at the 2003 amputee championships in Helsinki, and the 2004 and 2005 world championships in Prague. It was truly amazing to be a part of such a terrific program.

I would have loved to have continued with them even longer, but it just wasn't possible. As is the case with so many amateur sports in Canada, the funding just isn't there to make it a career and I had too many responsibilities and other things on the go to make it all work.

But I will never forget my time with these great players and having a chance to coach and work with them. These guys were perfect examples of never giving up – even being amputees wasn't enough to stop them from pursuing their passions at a high level. I am forever grateful for the chance I had to work with them for as long as I did.

CHAPTER 14

GETTING FUNDED

A key moment for the sport of sledge hockey came in March of 2005. Hockey Canada had its annual general meeting in Thunder Bay and the pressure was ramping up for us to try and get sledge hockey funded.

The head of sledge hockey Dean Delaurier told me point blank that "we can't continue to Torino paying our own expenses." In other words, we had to get some funding from Hockey Canada or else the cost of just getting to the Olympics was going to be too high for our players alone to bear. The always rising costs would make it prohibitive for anyone to continue playing our sport on the international level.

I knew that first hand. I was one of the players after all.

Keep in mind that I had always been the "spokesman" for our sport. I was the guy doing the media blitzes, speaking at events, always promoting and pleading our case. I even got Don Cherry to talk about us on Hockey Night in Canada. I was happy to do it – I loved to talk! – and this coming AGM in Thunder Bay was a make it or break it kind of meeting for sledge hockey.

We had to convince Hockey Canada it was time to properly fund our sport or our future Olympic participation would be very much in doubt. It was just as simple as that.

Greg Lagace of Sled Hockey of Canada told me "Rosey, you do the pitch" that had to be made to the Hockey Canada executive.

OK, now I love to talk as you know, but this was a real pressure cooker for me. So much was riding on this one pitch. I sure wasn't ready to give up my Olympic dreams, and I so badly wanted sledge hockey to get the funding it deserved, but there was a lot of competition from other disabled sports to get that funding.

Blind hockey, deaf hockey, roller hockey…the list was long of sports that wanted that desperately needed Hockey Canada funding. But I agreed to go to Thunder Bay and be the voice of the sledge hockey pitch.

I was sweating heading into that AGM boy. There were a lot of high profile hockey people in that room. I was just some guy and I'm sitting next to people like Canadian woman's hockey icon Cassie Campbell and former NHL great Steve Larmer. It was pretty intimidating.

But despite being nervous I took some deep breaths and made our pitch.

It worked. Sledge hockey got its funding.

I'm a bit of a ham, so I just told my story, how much it meant to me and my teammates to be able to represent Canada on the international stage. I put my sales hat on; you have to make people fall in love with your situation and tug at their heartstrings if they are going to give you their money and not give it to somebody else.

I told that AGM it had the opportunity to make the dreams of so many disabled athletes come true in the same city where the great Terry Fox ended his Marathon of Hope. Our dreams and Terry's dreams would live on, I told them, if they would fund us.

Their decision changed the lives of a lot of people. We no longer had to pay our own way to represent our country on the world stage. I was proud to be a part of making that happen.

CHAPTER 15

MAX'S FALL

I was certainly making progress in my hockey life during this time period. I was working my way into being the number one goalie and ticking another item off my goals list I had set years earlier, and now we'd be getting our expenses paid and a monthly honorarium from Hockey Canada to boot thanks to our successful pitch.

As all of this was happening my "non-hockey life" wasn't making much progress. In fact it was only getting worse.

My wife was still carrying the bulk of the financial load for our family, but I was at least earning some money from playing. I'd also started making a few dollars doing motivational speaking, which much later on became a successful enterprise for me.

Giving talks wasn't something that I had set out deliberately to get into, it just came about I guess. Just after I lost my leg, I was working with Shane Smith at Variety Village if you recall from earlier in the book.

Shane wanted me to talk to young kids and encourage them, to show them that life did go on after an amputation, and I was happy to do so. The best way to take the focus off your own problems is to help somebody focus on theirs, and that's what I started doing more and more.

I started doing the odd talk to groups, looking to encourage other people, and I did them for nothing. As time went on they were very well received and I started getting asked more and more often. In 2004 I did one at a school and received $500 which I was pretty grateful for at the time.

As the years went on I developed a speaking career but it basically evolved from my desire to help other people and find ways to encourage them, which I had done a lot of for a long time without making any money at it. My ability to talk and tell a story certainly paid off at the 2005 Hockey Canada AGM, and it certainly eventually paid off for me as a motivational speaker, but that didn't really happen until much later on.

My personal life was still quite rocky during many of these years. I was getting to be a bit well known due to my constant travel and promotion of sledge hockey, but fame doesn't pay any bills and it also meant I was never home. My family was never a top priority for me, it always played second fiddle to my hockey career and that is never a good thing.

I also still had Max Birbraer in my life. He also remained more important to me than my own family.

Earlier on I talked about meeting Max at the 1997 World Under-18 tournament. I used the word "obsession" while talking about trying to help get him a pro hockey career. While I was dealing with my leg amputation in 1999, the Team Canada situation in the early 2000s, my job and then departure at Benjamin's and my shaky home life - I was also still dealing with Max.

As I mentioned I basically went to all of his games when he played in the AHL, either driving eight hours to Albany or taking a Greyhound bus. I even moved in with him at one point, and continued mentoring him in the several years that followed, even after giving him to Brad Robbins to manage when I realized he'd be better off with him.

Joe Arfin was helping me all he could – and I really appreciated his dedication to helping Max succeed as well – but I was still spending way too much time on his life than I should have been, there's no doubt about that.

So I am a husband and father, a Team Canada athlete, and I am still very much involved in Max's life. My health is terrible during most of those years and I am being pulled in a thousand different directions at once.

I admit it – I was a bit of mess. And unfortunately, Max's crack at the big time was coming to an end at the same time.

He had tremendous potential to be an NHL player, but it never came to fruition for him for whatever reason. It isn't easy for anybody to make a career in the National Hockey League, no matter how good a player you are, and eventually when his contract was expiring with Albany, New Jersey General Manager Lou Lamoriello wound up releasing him.

The Los Angeles Kings picked him up, but he had gone from a pretty highly regarded prospect to just another player by that point, eventually winding up in the Central Hockey League in Laredo, Texas.

He spent time with the Devils, in the Kings organization and later had a look with the Florida Panthers, but he never played a game in the National Hockey League, so my dreams of cashing in if he ever signed a big contract never came to pass. Still, I don't regret the time and money I spent on him.

I loved the kid. Still do. And despite not making it in the NHL, he eventually made his way to Cardiff, England, and recently retired after playing pro hockey for 20 years, enjoying a very good run. He wound up playing 164 games in the AHL and was able to earn a living from the game, playing pro hockey elsewhere in the world, for a long time after his time in North America was up.

We still stay in touch to this day. We make a point of always talking on Father's Day and I have a tattoo on my right arm with two hockey sticks and the number 25, with the slogan "Brothers forever" written in Hebrew. Max has the identical tattoo. Our first numbers playing hockey for both of us were 25, so we immortalized our relationship with identical tattoos – that is how tight we are.

So I do not regret all of the attention I gave to Max. But I do regret that I wasn't as good a father to my own kids as I was to Max. And that wasn't just the case from 1997 to 1999, when I basically followed Max around North America to watch him play, it was also the case during the early 2000s where I dedicated a lot of time to him as well.

The world knew me as Paul Rosen, sledge hockey player and spokesman, and as a budding motivational speaker. Max knew me as a surrogate father.

But my own kids didn't even really know me…I was never home and I was never there for them like I was for Max.

It was especially rough at home from the start of 2004 right up until the Torino Olympics as I was grasping to try and save things, and that really led to the final downfall of my marriage. I even contemplated suicide a few times that summer after the world championships.

Max had left for England by that point, his dreams (and mine) of an NHL career gone. He would turn his life around and play for many years around the world, but I missed him often and always regretted that he didn't achieve his ultimate dream.

Looking back on it now I don't know how I got through the years 2004 and 2005 with the crazy schedule, the health issues, the poor home life and the winding down of Max's career in North America.

While I impressed the country with my passionate plea for sledge hockey funding in 2005, my own life was in tatters a lot of time. Yet somehow I kept going, as another Olympic Games were on the horizon and I had to be there for Team Canada. And Max kept playing hockey, looking for ways to achieving at least a piece of his dream.

Max and I had something in common besides a tattoo I guess. We both never gave up.

CHAPTER 16

SECOND OLYMPICS

There was a new regime running Team Canada now as we got ready for the Torino Olympics in 2006. We also had Hockey Canada full funding which was great. But with full funding comes the full pressure to perform – when you are funded you are expected to win medals, not come in fourth place as we had the 2002 Olympics.

I was always "all in" in my desire to win and perform as a sledge hockey player, but I now really went to another level. I started heavy training, going to the gym every day to workout. We're making about $1,500 a month now and there was an education package included for the younger players, so it was a pretty sweet deal compared to the NOTHING we had been getting before.

I felt the added pressure, but I had always felt pressure to some degree, always wanting to be at my best whenever I was wearing a Team Canada jersey. That's just the way I was wired. I could see that under Coach Snyder we were starting to jell and there was definitely much more structure to the program than there was prior to his coming on board. That was a very positive sign.

We were at a tournament in October of 2005 in Japan that gave an indication of how good we could be. We played six games and I had six shutouts, and it was a real stepping stone for us to reassert ourselves as a top sledge hockey country. It was a real confidence booster for everyone. We were so dominant.

Snyder was the reason. He brought a plan and a program and instilled some discipline where there had been none prior. Things were looking up, but there was still a lot of work to do before Torino.

The last training camp took place in Calgary in February as we got ready for the Games. I was really feeling the pressure to perform. Not only that, I had to stop the puck and be the team spokesman at the same time as always of course.

Let me be totally honest again – I didn't shy away from the PR responsibility. I loved talking. The limelight was kind of cool. But that still didn't make it any easier on me, as I was the guy always out there in front of the cameras and therefore if we didn't win, it would be me the fingers would be pointed at.

We got a ton of publicity leading up to the Olympics. While I was in Toronto I was interviewed by Scott Oake right at ice level on Hockey Night in Canada. Don Cherry and Ron McLean interviewed me during training camp in Calgary on CBC. I told them simply "It's a business trip, we're going to win a gold medal."

Brave words, but just one problem with them; we were only ranked number four in the world and even though the signs were encouraging leading into the Games, we weren't considered the clear favorites that I was telling everyone we should be.

Still, it was an exciting time despite the pressure. Our training camp wrapped up in Calgary and we headed for the Paralympics in Torino. I couldn't wait to get there; being able to just concentrate on playing would be easier than training and having to hype the whole event up for publicity purposes. The regular Olympic Games don't need hype. The Paralympics can always use publicity, and it was my job to deliver it on behalf of sledge hockey.

The pressure only got worse. Hockey Canada's Bob Nicholson pulled me aside in Torino one day and told me how it was so important for us to win because of the funding we had been given. Over the long run funding is based on results and it is given to remove all excuses – there would be none accepted if we couldn't win this time.

The fact that the men's hockey team had flamed out and finished seventh in the Olympics sure didn't help matters (although the women did bring home the gold and thank God that they did!).

We were assigned Team Canada's dressing room. I was sitting in the same stall that Martin Brodeur had. Now that's pressure my friends.

Even though things were not good in my home life, I arranged for my family to come to Torino and witness the Games. They were in the stands watching. The whole world was watching as we got ready to go after a gold medal.

The 2006 Torino Olympics turned out to be the greatest moment of my playing career – but they also led to the worst moment of my personal life.

Before I continue talking about Torino, I want to say a few things here about coach Jeff's nephew Dan Snyder.

While playing for the Atlanta Thrashers in 2003, Dan Snyder was killed in a car crash. The car was driven by his teammate Dany Heatley. It was such a tragic event and made headlines around the world.

Heatley was charged with vehicular homicide, driving too fast for conditions, failure to maintain a lane, and speeding. He could have received up to 15 years in prison, but was eventually sentenced to three years' probation and ordered to give 150 speeches on the dangers of speeding and pay $25,000 to Fulton Court for the cost of the investigation of the crash.

The lighter sentence was primarily due to the forgiveness of Snyder's parents and family. They did not want to see Heatley go to prison, which tells you a lot about the kind of people the Snyders are.

Dan's funeral was attended by every member of the Owen Sound Platers (his junior team) and the Atlanta Thrashers, along with all of us on Team Canada's sledge hockey team. His memory became a rallying cry for us at the Olympics, as we "circulated the chain" in his honor.

Coach Snyder talked to us about his nephew's legacy, and the importance of staying together as a team no matter what. He made a chain with 22 links in it (15 players and seven staff), and said each of us was a link in that chain.

We were all asked to name a person we were dedicating this tournament to (for me it was my Dad), and we all circled around and held that chain as a sign of team unity. We then talked about how we were all important to one another. If one link in the chain breaks, the whole chain breaks.

It was one of the most emotional events I have ever been a part of. I still have my link of that chain and I use it in every motivational talk I give. We were 15 hearts, one heartbeat…that was our slogan. I still get chills thinking about the impact of that memory.

After such an emotional ceremony, we were so ready to go. It was time to go out there and win a gold medal…for all of us.

◼ ◼ ◼

It was finally time for my second Olympics. So many things had changed in the four years since the 2002 Games in Salt Lake City.

I was an established veteran on the team by now, and playing for Team Canada is all that mattered in my life. I was so involved in playing and promoting the team that I had to leave the job I loved at Benjamin's, so I was "all in" during these Olympic Games. I had brought my whole family to see this and I was determined we were going to win this time around.

I'm now also 46 years old. I'm telling the younger players to treat this like it was a business trip – we were here to do one thing and one thing only; that's win a gold medal.

We had built up some confidence with some good results in tournaments prior to Torino, but after finishing fourth in 2002, we had some serious improvements to make if we were going to win that gold.

The tournament started with an easy game. We played Italy and won 13-0. We were incredibly dominant, so much so that I think I fell asleep twice during that game! I faced three shots all night and there was no doubt after that opening performance we were going to be a force to be reckoned with this time around.

We then beat the highly regarded Swedes 3-0, as I posted another shutout. We were sky high, and looked to be unstoppable…until we ran into Norway in our third game.

Norway was an excellent team and on this particular night, they were just better than we were. No excuses. We were trailing 4-1 and considering where we were in the tournament, and the score of the game, it made sense for us to pull me and let our back-up Benny St.Amode get some playing time in the Olympics.

I was having none of that. Being lifted would have just been too much for my ego.

I pleaded with Snyder to let me finish the game. "Keep me in and I promise you, I won't give up another goal in the tournament," I remember telling him. In my mind I just had to play the rest of that game.

I was adamant. I even told my back-up Benny to his face that he wasn't going into the game, I was staying in and that was that.

Time for more honesty here – that was a really stupid thing to do. I was prick.

I was at the peak of my career as a sledge hockey goalie, but I was a terrible teammate to do that, especially at that point in the game and the tournament. There was no reason for me to stay in the game, and I regret acting that way.

I make no excuses for it now; but the combination of my ego, the pressure I was feeling and my personal lifestyle (I was still a drug and alcohol abuser) just got to me I suppose.

I lived for the fame of being a Team Canada goalie. Every time I was recognized it just fed my ego. I couldn't stand the thought of being pulled from a game.

I remember during the tournament one night I took my mother and father-in-law to dinner. After dinner I went back to the athlete's village and my family took a cab back to their hotel.

All of the family members were given lanyards to wear identifying them as being with the Olympics so they could travel around easier. The driver noticed them and started talking about how he'd watched a Team Canada sledge hockey game, and that the Canadian goalie was so great, fans were chanting his name "Rosey!" over and over. My family beamed with pride, they all told me. Hearing that kind of story only stroked my ego more.

My win at all costs attitude helped me become the goalie I was; I have no doubt about that. But I became as dependent on getting that attention and being the great Paul Rosen the goalie as I was dependent on narcotics and alcohol when I wasn't playing to get through the day. There was no middle ground for me, and it had to be my way or the highway…in everything.

So I stayed in the game. They didn't score again in the third period, so we lost 4-1.

We were human after all. I was human after all. After two shutouts I had been lit up a bit. And I had made matters worse by being an ass and not letting myself get pulled, and then boldly saying I wouldn't give up another goal.

There was pressure before that Norway game, but now it was frankly just ridiculous. And I had nobody to blame but myself for that.

▣ ▣ ▣

Next up is the semi-final. We are playing Germany, another very strong team. I had basically guaranteed a shutout, as I begged to be kept in against Norway by flatly stating I wouldn't give up another goal in the tournament if they kept me in there.

Final score of the semi-final game: Canada 5, Germany 0. I was an ass, but I at least did back up my promise by not allowing a goal.

We were onto the gold medal game. We were one game away from winning it all. Our opponents would again be Norway, the team that had beaten us rather handily just a few days prior.

Look, I am not going to pretend that sledge hockey means as much to Canadians as the Olympic tournament featuring NHLers does. But there were a lot of eyes on us and a lot of expectations, especially after the men's team's poor performance in the Olympics. The game was televised, there was a great crowd on hand, and we were feeling the pressure big time. The fact I was acting the way I was certainly didn't help the cause either.

Before the game we had an important message sent to us. As we were having our morning breakfast waiting for the game to start, we were told "Somebody wants to say hello to you."

On a speaker phone then comes the voice of Wayne Gretzky.

He gave us an inspiring speech, reminding us of how important teammates are to each other and how we were all connected in the pursuit of this gold medal. It was a beautiful moment and just what we needed. It wasn't all about "me" after all – it was about all of "us" in this together.

We were sky high after that chat. I was never more sure we were going to win a game than I was on that day.

We got on the ice and the place was going crazy. I looked over at one of Norway's top players and blew him a kiss. It drove him nuts! He promptly goes after Westlake just after the game starts and takes a penalty, and we are off to the races already. We were in their heads.

It was our day and it was our time. We scored just over a minute into the game, and had a 2-0 lead after two periods. During the second intermission, I told the team "Boys, we've got this gold medal. This moment we will have the rest of our lives."

The final 30 seconds ticked down. We added another goal with four seconds left and won 3-0.

We were gold medal winners.

I had kept up my end of the bargain that I made to not be pulled in that first game against Norway. I did not allow another goal after that moment, and the team played tremendous hockey in front of me. It had been a long, trying road but we were deserving gold medal winners. All of the hard work had paid off.

It was just pandemonium after that final siren.

Shortly after we won, Don Cherry placed a call to me from Coach's Corner on Hockey Night in Canada, right on live national TV. I will never forget that one minute interview.

Craig Campbell grabbed my mask. He wanted for the Hockey Hall of Fame. There was another goal of mine from way back accomplished – I would have some sort of presence in the Hockey Hall of Fame after all. What a thrill that was, to know my mask was going to be in the Hall.

We didn't leave that dressing room until maybe 5 in the morning the next day. We had thousands of cans of beers in that arena! (As an aside, that arena was built just for the Olympic Games. It was constructed and ready in time, and was torn down right after, which is kind of amazing when you think about it.)

Our dressing room was a wild place that night. The entire Italian team came in we really liked those guys; in fact anybody we liked was welcomed to come in, and we all had a few beers that night let me tell you. It was an amazing celebration.

And of course I had to take a drug test. It was the Olympics after all. When I say "of course I" - there was never any doubt that I would be one of the athletes signaled out for testing. I passed it, which was no surprise to anybody, because I must have had RANDOM written on my birth certificate somewhere!

I must have been "random" tested 11 times at various points in my career, far more than any of my other teammates. I was either really unlucky or somebody must have thought I was on a performance enhancing substance of some kind during my career. But it was all good, I didn't really care and I knew that I was clean.

I also knew, and we all knew, we'd have that gold medal forever. Nothing was ever going to change that and we were all delirious as a result. What a great night that was!

The next couple of days were just crazy, but in a terrific kind of way. We had numerous team dinners and wound up staying a few days longer. When we arrived back home at Pearson International Airport in Toronto, the crowd there to greet us was just great. We had brought home the first gold medal from a hockey team at the Paralympics to Canada and it was just an amazing feeling.

My mask was going to be in the Hockey Hall of Fame, which was a pretty cool thing to know. I felt like a million dollars – we had done what we all set out to do and we were flying high after those Games were over.

At that point in 2006, it was the best year of my life. Before the year was over though, it would also become the worst year of my life.

CHAPTER 17

MARRIAGE ENDS

I said earlier that prior to the 2006 Games; things weren't very good at home. That was an understatement actually.

I was spending more and more time away from home before the Olympics and when we returned after that fantastic experience, it only got worse. I was NEVER home after that.

Paul Rosen was now a bit of a celebrity, and did that ever stroke my ego. I came back from the Olympics with a gold medal after all – which went great along with my gold medal mouth.

Winning a gold medal did a lot for my public speaking career, as I now had another great story to tell and a gold medal to show off. I had hooked up with The Ad Lib Group in 2003 and they started getting a lot more offers for me to speak. That group's name was perfect for me by the way – all I ever did was ad lib. I spoke from the heart and my talks became more and more popular.

I kept right on with my training; I never let up for second. We were being paid $1,500 monthly now and I made sure Hockey Canada got their money's worth out of me. The 2007 World Cup was coming up in Kelowna, B.C. and we'd be facing rivals Norway, the United States and Germany again. They'd want some revenge from the Paralympics, so I was going to be sure I was ready. We also continued playing in various tournaments all over the place.

I totally ignored my family life as a result of all this new found celebrity. I was a very poor husband and father.

My youngest daughter Nikki really struck a nerve with me when she told me that I "cared about other people more than you care about us." That really hurt – but she was right. That had been the case for almost a decade actually, but now it was even more so. I missed her birthday that year, and that really started the downfall of our relationship.

I was doing really well financially ironically enough, but my marriage was also clearly falling apart. My wife had stuck by me for so long, putting up with all my drama and all my travels, and basically had raised the kids herself. We had split up several times, had many fights, but she always gave me second chances after I pleaded with her that I'd be a better father and husband.

In late 2006, she'd finally had enough. We split up for good.

It devastated me, and while my hockey career and speaking career were going full throttle by now, my personal life was completely off the rails.

I was really drinking hard by this point, and popping any pill I could get my hands on. I just couldn't come to grips with my problems at home. Later on in my life Alcohol Anonymous would wind up saving me, but back then I wasn't looking for help from anyone.

I was contemplating suicide all the time. I really was a mess, and on January 7, 2007 I left home for the final time and moved in with Brad Robbins and his family. It was a new low for me.

Life is full of ups and downs…especially mine I guess. I went from the exhilarating high of winning a gold medal at the Olympics in early 2006 to the extreme low of losing my family by the time the year was out. By early 2007 I had to move in with a friend.

I had a gold medal. I had a speaking career. I was better off financially. But I had a paid a high price for all that. The price I paid was losing my family.

CHAPTER 18

FAMILY TRAGEDY

Even when it is full of ups and downs, life goes on. My life went on in 2007 without my wife and family being with me.

All my life consisted of at that point was hockey. I lived for Team Canada. Nothing else mattered. Fortunately for me, the hockey was still going pretty well.

It's March 17, 2007, and it's time for the gold medal game at the World Cup in Kelowna. We had a great tournament and were poised to win another world championship to go along with our Paralympic gold.

I get a phone call before the final game that morning…my ex-wife Cheryl's mother had passed away. She was a wonderful person well loved by her kids.

My family wanted me to come back home right away and help deal with this sad tragedy. Here's how I reacted to that news.

I hung up on them and then got back on the phone and contacted Benjamin's. They would look after the arrangements. I didn't care about my family's wishes that I be with them. We had the gold medal game to play. I'm not going anywhere.

That reaction to Cheryl's mother's passing pretty much describes what my mindset was like during this time period. It is painful for me to remember this, but I've said all along in this book that I'm going to be honest so here goes – I didn't give a f*&k about my family's wishes at that point. The most important thing in the world to me was sledge hockey, not them.

After making the arrangements for her with Benjamin's, I went about the business of getting ready for the game like nothing had happened. Part of my game day preparation was taking six Oxycodones before we headed out on the ice. That's the state I was in.

My teammates felt badly for me when they heard the news…so much so we wore black arm bands in her memory. They basically showed more compassion for her than I was showing; I was just strung out and all I wanted to focus on was winning a game.

This particular game was against Norway and the World Cup was at stake. We hated them and they hated us, and I for one thrived on the fact that they hated me. I put all thoughts of family aside and went out to win the game.

The place was absolutely packed. If the fire department was there they would have closed the place down for being over-capacity. It was rematch of the 2006 Games final and it was extremely intense right from the start.

The game was scoreless and went into overtime. I stopped a breakaway in the first minute with a terrific save, and made a pass up the ice. We score with 37 seconds gone in overtime and win the game 1-0. I get a shutout and an assist on the game-winning goal.

We are world champions. We celebrate madly on the ice. My teammates are filled with joy.

I felt like a piece of dog shit.

What I had done hit me hard right as we celebrated that victory. I chose Team Canada over my own family, and I was so far gone it didn't even bother me until after the game was over. To the world I was a goaltending star, a motivational speaker, a great guy…but I sure didn't feel like any of those things then.

I knew that I was coming home from that tournament with nothing to come home to. I had moved out of Brad's home by then and was living in a small apartment by myself. Nobody in my family wanted to talk to me, especially after the way I had acted about Cheryl's mother dying and my refusal to even consider coming back home right away to help them with the arrangements in person.

We had another gold medal. Big deal. On the ice I was a champion once again, but off the ice I was just a loser in my own mind.

Everybody loved Rosey in those days – except the people who mattered most to me. I had never felt so alone.

CHAPTER 19

MEDAL STOLEN

I might have felt alone, but I was in the spotlight more and more after the gold medal at the 2006 Olympics and another gold medal at the 2007 World Cup.

I was doing a lot of speaking engagements and autograph sessions and the like, so that part of my life was going quite well actually. And funny enough, a theft resulted in my national popularity soaring to the greatest heights in February, 2007.

During this time I had started being involved with my great friend Kerry Goulet's Stop Concussions project, and his Shoot for a Cure charity. We were at Downsview Park one Saturday for an autograph session and were taking a lot of photos and having some fun for a good cause.

Whenever an event like this came around, I turned it on. I was Mr. Happiness. The world had no idea what my true state of mind was, since I was always smiling when "the lights were on" in any capacity.

I had the Paralympic gold medal with me that day that I had won on March 18, 2006, which was naturally my most prized possession. I brought it to all my talks and people enjoyed being able to see and hold it whenever I made a public appearance.

Cheryl Pounder from the Canadian women's hockey team was also there, as were a lot of other noted hockey people. Cheryl also had her gold medal with her and we posed for pictures with fans throughout the day. It was nice.

It was getting time to wrap up for the day, and I was having a good chat with the late Bob Probert, just shooting the breeze, when Cheryl started packing everything up. She came up to Probert and I while we were talking.

"Rosey, where's your gold medal?" she said to me.

"Its right next to yours on the table," I told her, continuing my chat with Probert.

"It's not there," Cheryl told me.

Oh. My. God.

I went into absolute panic mode. We locked the park down and began a frantic search, looking everywhere inside that place for my medal. We searched that place up and down for what seemed like hours.

It was gone.

We didn't have any real security at these kind of events, and our medals were on a table in front of us for most of the day, unless we picked them up to pose for pictures or let somebody have the fun of holding it.

Somebody had obviously stolen it while we weren't paying attention and there was no security to stop them. I was crushed.

Who would steal such a personal item like that, right from under our noses, at a charity event for God's sake? Maybe a kid took it not knowing any better, but whatever the case, my precious gold medal was missing.

Cheryl felt awful, and she immediately got on the phone to her former teammate Cassie Campbell. Cassie was married to Brad Pascal of Hockey Canada, who had been heavily involved with our sledge hockey program right from the start, to tell him what had happened.

Cassie then made a few more phone calls and got in touch with Hockey Night in Canada. On his Coach's Corner segment that night on CBC, Don Cherry made a nationally broadcast plea for whoever took my medal to return it.

Don (bless his heart for doing so) went on a real rant, telling the story to the millions of viewers he had and demanding that "the rats who took Rosey's medal" should just drop it in a mailbox and send it back to me. This was apprehensible, he told the country.

It was great of him to do it, but there was no consoling me that weekend. I went home Saturday night and spent the rest of the weekend in total shock. I couldn't believe what had happened.

I shook off my bitter disappointment on Monday however, and became determined to get my medal back; although I knew in my mind any attempt to do so was probably a long shot. That week turned out to be just crazy, from Monday to Friday.

Don's profile was enormous of course, and the rest of the media responded to his comments on Coach's Corner by contacting me for interviews. I was on CTV's Canada AM twice that week, and I did interview after interview with media outlets from everywhere pleading for my medal to be returned.

I was devastated. In the mental state I was in, this was an especially tough loss to bear. I lived for my hockey and that gold medal was everything to me. I prayed that the appeals I was launching would lead to its return, but in the back of my mind I figured my medal was gone forever.

What happened next was nothing short of amazing.

One week to the day it was stolen, I received a call from 32 Division. I was told they had my medal.

I couldn't believe it! I rushed to the station along with Michael Abramson, who was my speaking agent at the time from the Ad Lib Group, absolutely delighted that somehow my medal had been found.

When we got to the precinct, the parking lot was jammed! There were trucks and cars from every media outlet you can imagine, all of whom wanted to capture the story of the return of my medal for their news channels.

My joy was tempered a bit when I made my way inside. The police were not amused.

"This is just a medal, not a murder case," one officer told the media throng outside. I was ushered into an office and was basically interrogated by some officers about the whole situation.

I don't know if they thought maybe I had staged the event and was just looking for publicity – which I was definitely not doing – but they really grilled me with questions. I just wanted to get my medal and get the hell out of there!

After a rather long series of questions, the police told me that the medal had been dropped into a mailbox and made its way to Canada Post's Eastern Avenue central sorting area.

Whoever had stolen the medal had followed Don Cherry's advice to the letter – they just tossed it into a mailbox with no envelope! That certainly shows the power Don wielded in those days, and I'll be forever grateful he used his pulpit to help me.

The police brought out my medal. The ribbon looked like it had been chewed on by a dog, it was so tattered from the travels it had made, but it wasn't damaged beyond that. My hands shook when the officers handed it back to me.

We wound never find out who had stolen it, since so many sets of fingerprints were on it by the time the cops received it, and there was no other evidence. But my medal had been returned to me thanks to Grapes, and that's all I really cared about.

I then went out into the parking lot and was met by the media throng who recorded my happy reunion with my medal. I will tell you this though – the police were really pissed. I talked to the reporters as quickly as I could so they'd clear the area, and Michael and I left with the medal around my chest.

Michael was smiling ear to ear from the time we drove up to the station until the time we left it.

"This is going to make your speaking career take off," he told me. "Everybody is going to want to see the stolen gold medal!"

I really didn't pay attention to his comment or really care at that point; I just wanted my medal back. But Michael sure turned out to be right.

The next year and half was the absolute height of my speaking career, it was just insane the number of offers that came in to us. The media exposure I got from such a terrible theft happening to me wound up leading to a great period for me business-wise. It just goes to show you that good things can come from bad. For the next 18 months or so, I was busier than ever because everybody wanted to see Paul Rosen's stolen gold medal…so we may as well let him talk to us!

I tell that story at all my speaking engagements to this day. And I say here now to the police who had to put up with the ruckus that day – I'm so sorry for the trouble I caused.

However it sure made for a great story!

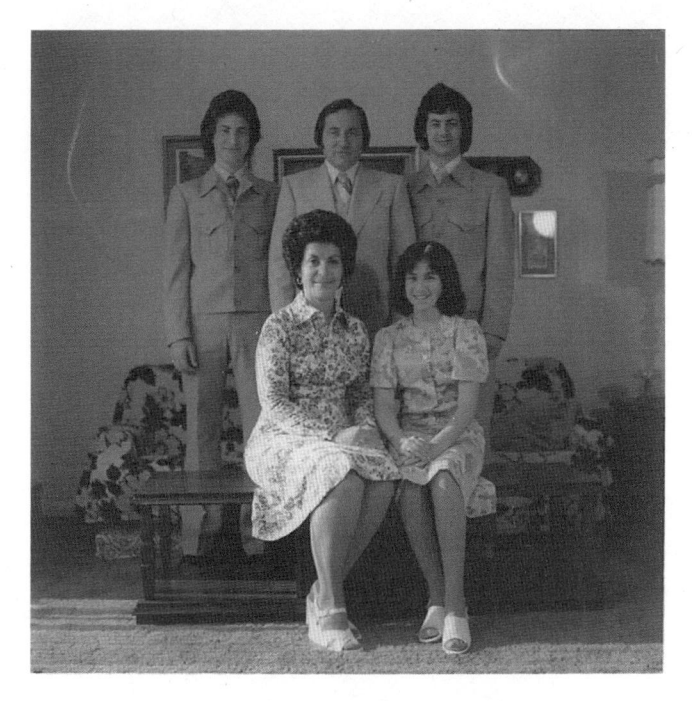

The traditional family pic of my siblings and parents, showing off in our Sunday bests!

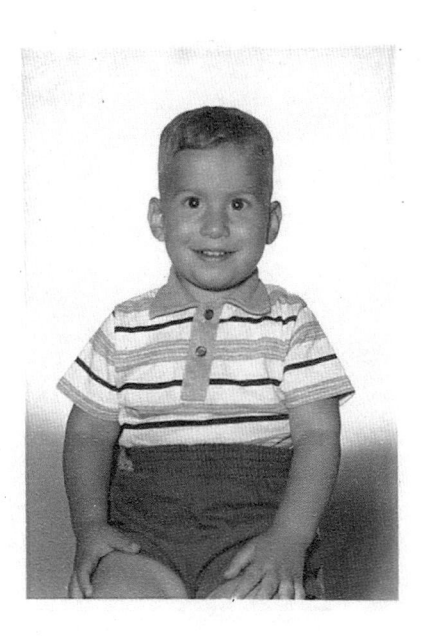

Hard to believe but I am just two years old in this picture.

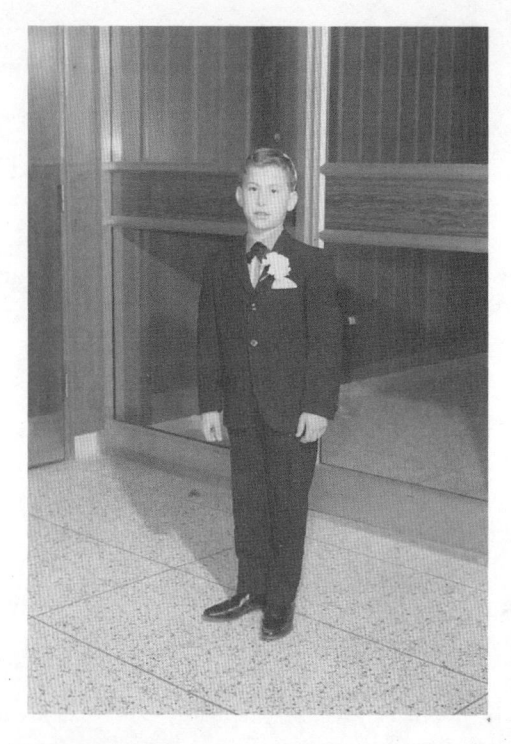

I'm 9 years old here at my brother's Bar Mitzvah in 1969.

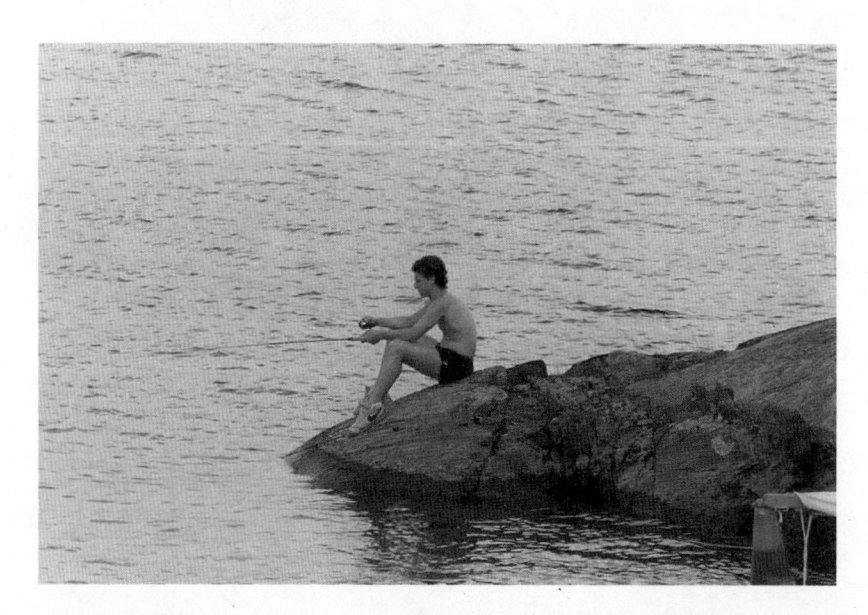

Here at 17 at the family cottage in 1977, the first time I contemplated killing myself.

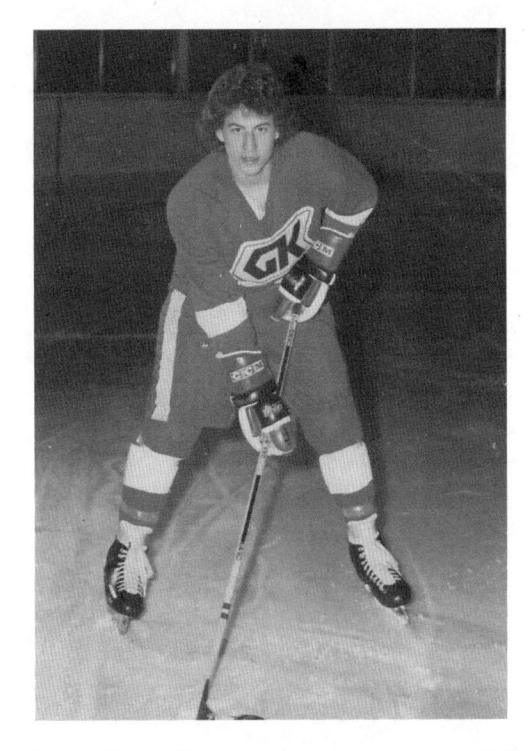

With the Thornhill midgets minor hockey team in 1975.

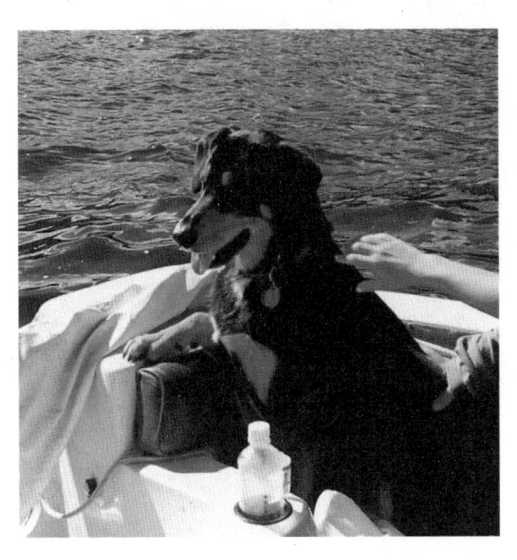

My beloved dog Gilly, named after close friend Paul Gillis of the Quebec Nordiques.

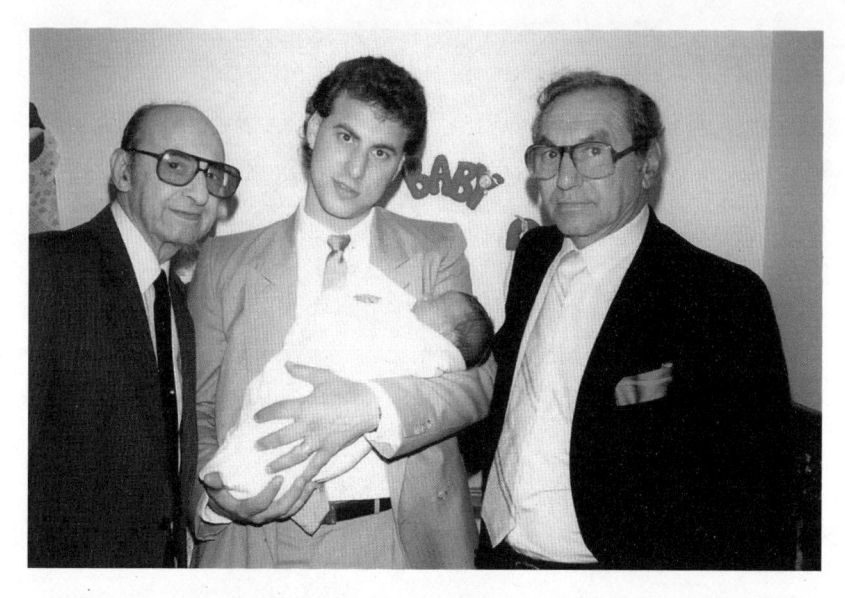

Four generations of Rosens. Holding my infant son with my grandfather Sid and father Ron.

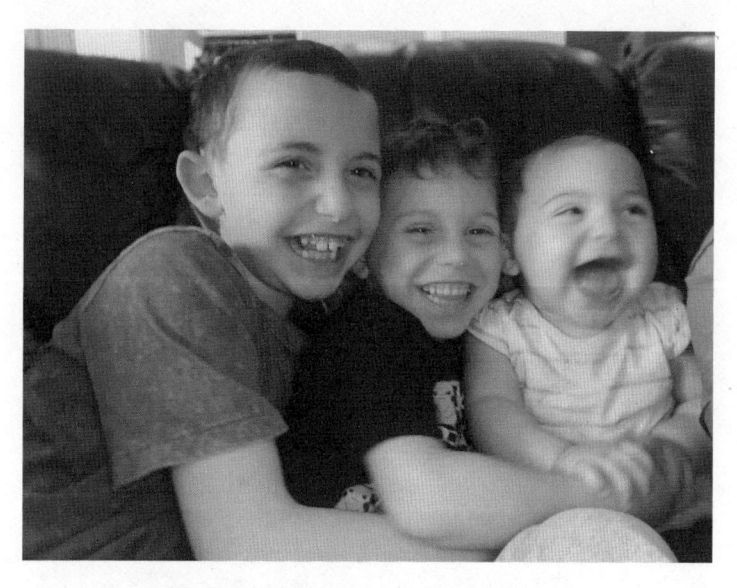

My terrific grandchildren Brody, Zac and Liv.

NEVER GIVE UP

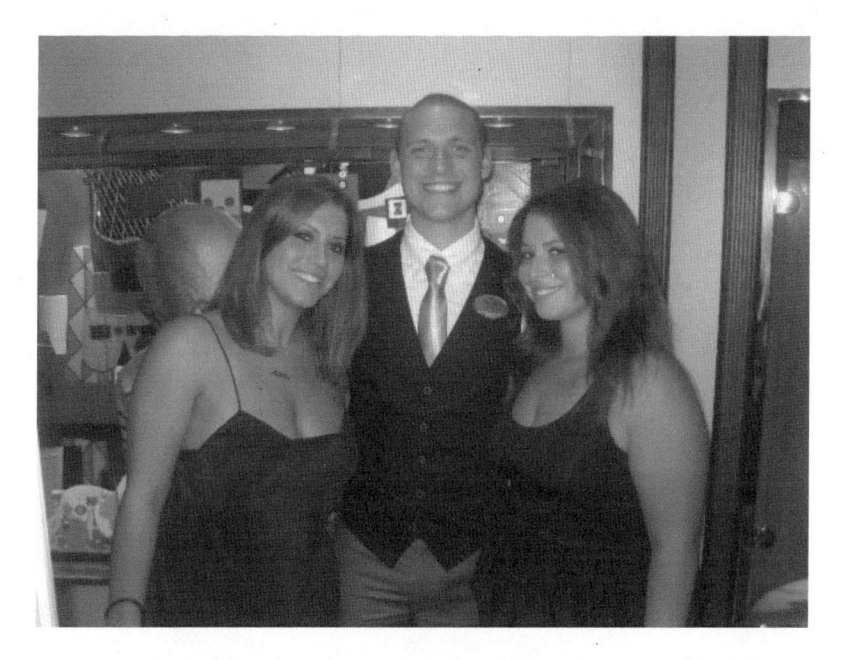

My son Sam working his job on a cruise ship with my daughters Nikki (left) and Stephanie (right).

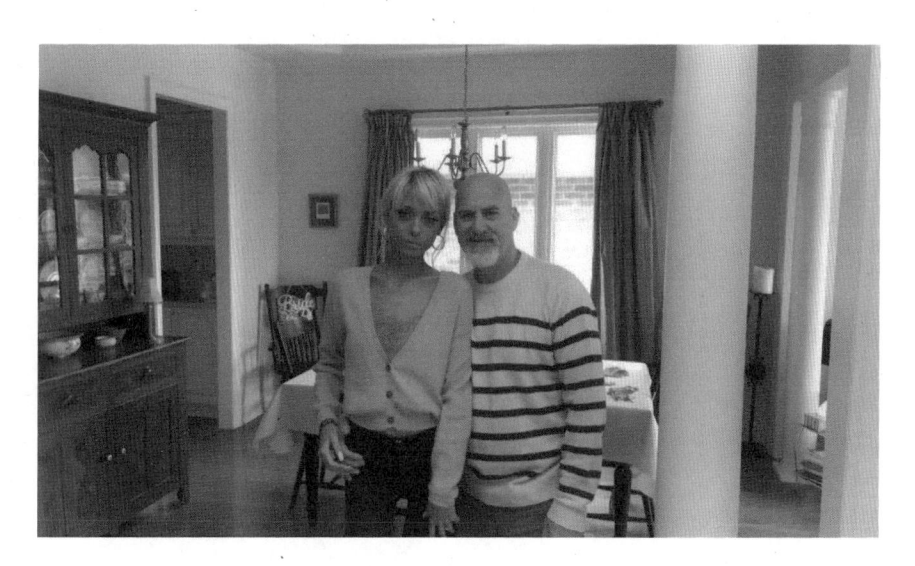

With the beautiful Arianna Markle.

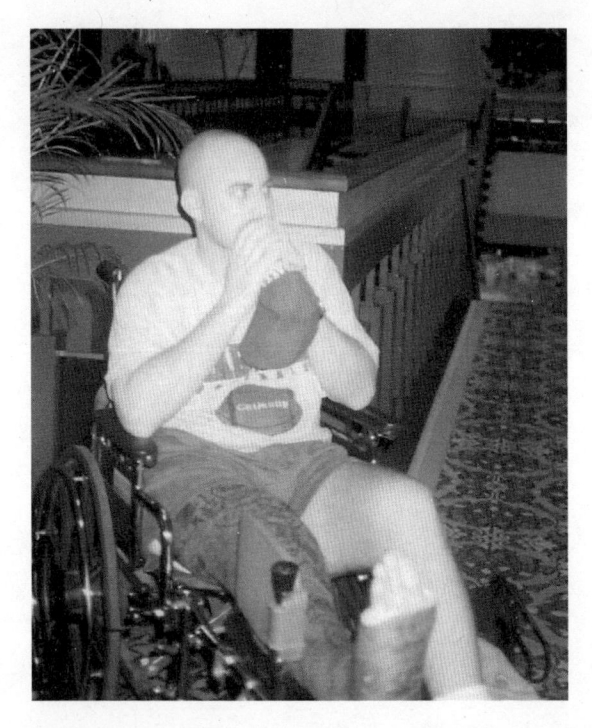

Watching my son at a dance competition in 1999, looking terrible. Several months later my leg is amputated.

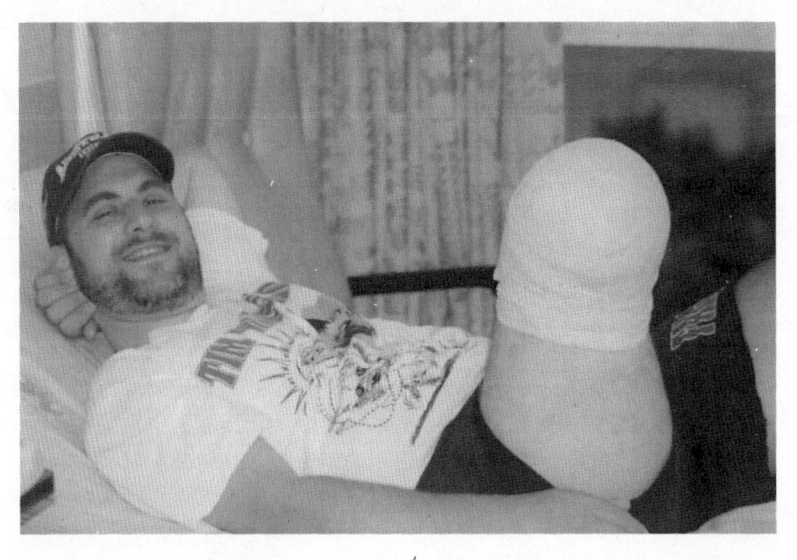

Just one day after my amputation in June, 1999 – smiling and ready to take on the world.

NEVER GIVE UP

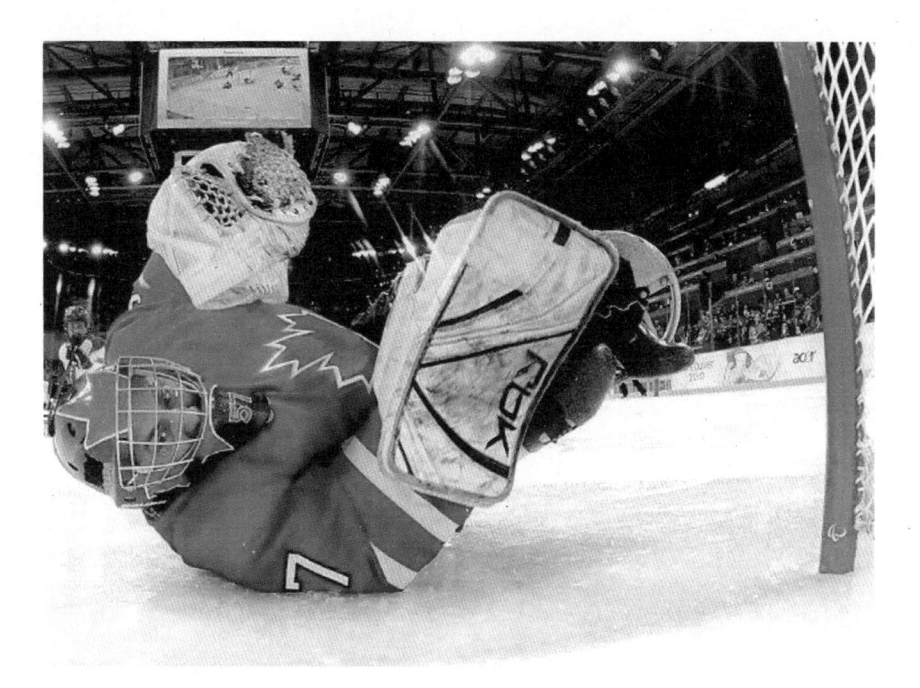

Vancouver 2010 Olympics, Game 1 versus Italy. We were so dominant I was dozing off and had to turn around and make a panic save after staring at the scoreboard! We won 5-0.

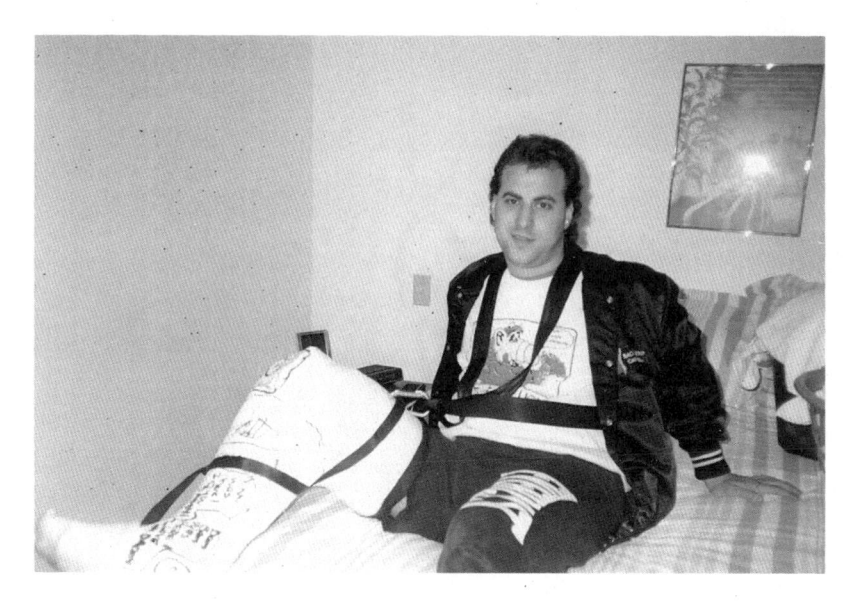

From the early 1980s after yet another one of the surgeries I had on my leg.

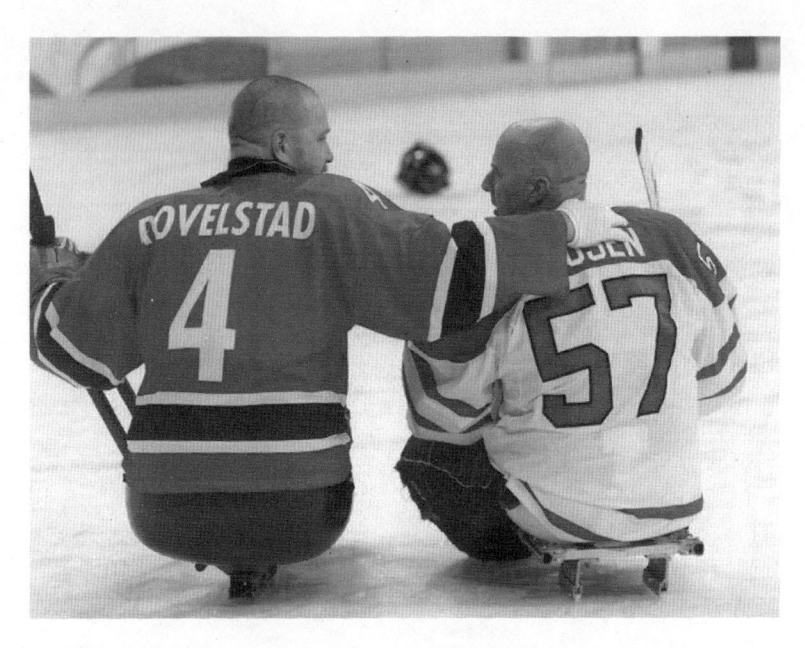

After the bronze medal game of the 2010 Olympics in Vancouver with Tommy Rovelstad. We were bitter rivals but it was the final game for both of us, so a chance to congratulate each other.

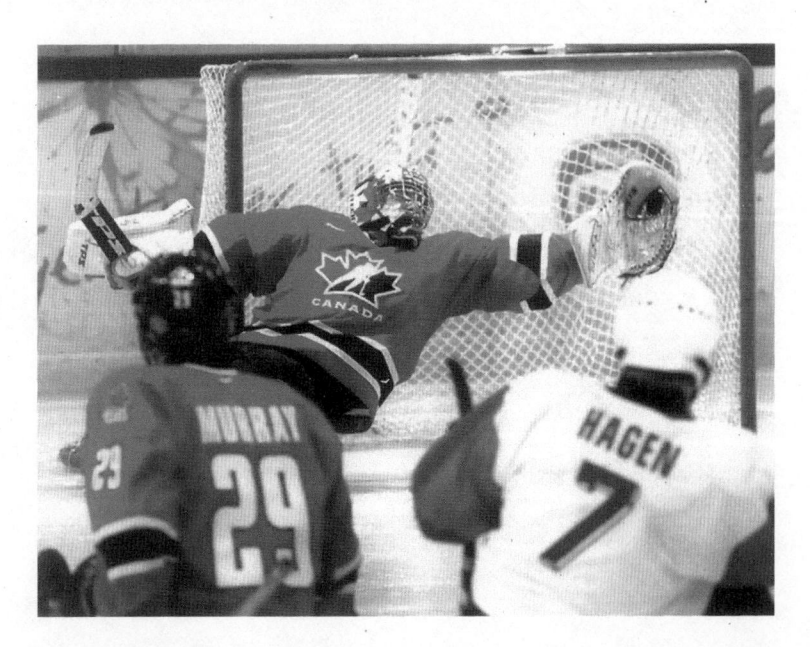

2008 World Championships in Boston; the picture that defines my career. We just call it THE SAVE!

CHAPTER 20

SITTING VOLLEYBALL

I want to include another story here about how I became one of the few athletes in Canadian Olympic or Paralympic history to have medals from two different sports, as that happened right in this time period.

So I've recovered my stolen gold medal as you've just read, my speaking career is now booming, but I'm still living in my small apartment in May of 2007.

Thank God I got busier with speaking in this time period, as I really needed the distraction away from my crumbling personal life. And that speaking boom led me to another sport in the most unusual way you can imagine.

I was invited to go to the University of Ottawa for a talk to a military group. I was always honored to be asked to do those; I have full respect for anything to do with the military. This one was for a group called Solider On, which is the American equivalent of our Wounded Warriors organization, another group I have supported in the past.

The goal of Solider On is to help returning veterans live better lives, and it raises funds to assist them. There is no better cause than that in my mind, so I was happy to drive up to Ottawa and speak with them at a meeting they were holding up there. It also got me out of my depressing apartment.

The talk went extremely well. I was well received and I was delighted to meet and talk with so many great people. Afterwards I was thanked and the organizers invited me to stay over another night as their guest at the hotel, instead of me driving all the way back home that night.

I thanked them, but my first thought was to decline their kind offer. As I've talked about earlier, when the light came on, I was on – but that didn't mean the light stayed on in my own personal life. When it was time to do a talk or do a broadcast, I was the Paul Rosen everybody knew and loved. As soon as it ended, I went back to my miserable personal existence.

So I was going to just say no thanks and drive back home right away. But then I thought – what am I rushing back to? I was only going to return to my little apartment and watch TV anyway, so I said I'd take them up on their offer and stay another night.

I really didn't have any other reason to stay another night in Ottawa except for the fact that it was better than going home. So I stayed another night at the hotel and the next day, with nothing special to do, I thought I'd just take a walk around the University of Ottawa campus. Maybe the Gee Gees sports teams were working out or something; I could go by and see them practice, give me something to do.

So I'm just wandering around the campus when I bump into Phil Allen, who was the head of the Canadian disabled volleyball team. He recognized me and came over and introduced himself and we had a nice chat.

He asked me what I was doing in Ottawa. I told him about my talk, and added that I was just killing some time walking around campus hoping to maybe see a university team practice or something before I headed home.

"Our sitting volleyball team is having a practice right now," Allen told me. "I'm sure they'd love it if you came by and said hello. Would you mind?"

I said sure. What else did I have to do? We walked over to the gym where they were meeting.

Full disclosure here – I had no idea what sitting volleyball was all about before I went into that gym. I had never paid attention to it before that day.

I was introduced to the team's captain and found out all about the team and the sport itself. Canada didn't have a very good team at that time, but they were going to go and compete at the Pan Am Games in Rio de Janerio later that year to gain some experience and help grow the sport.

I sat and watched them for a while and was pretty impressed with them and the way they played. They only had seven guys on the team, and five of them were under 24 years old.

They asked me if I'd ever played volleyball myself. I had. As I talked about earlier I was quite an athlete back in my younger days, and played high school volleyball.

"But that was in 1974!" I told them with a laugh.

"Get out here, let's see what you can do!" one of the players said to me.

Hell why not, I thought. This looks kind of fun. So right there and then in the gym, I took my artificial leg off and joined them to play a little sitting volleyball, just for fun. Spending a few hours fooling around in the gym sure beat going home in my mind.

A few months later I somehow found myself playing for Team Canada at the Pan Am Games in Rio! Honestly, it was just freaking amazing how it all unfolded.

I took to the sport right away, but what they liked about me was my veteran leadership. I became a bit of an instant leader with the younger players, as I'd played in two Paralympics by then and I knew what representing Canada on the international stage was all about.

I never really intended to stay with them for a long time – hell I was 47 years old by then, hadn't played volleyball in more than 30 years, and was heavily committed to the sledge hockey program of course.

But they were insistent that they wanted me to be a part of the team. They were short of players and would be in some trouble if anybody got injured, so one thing led to another and they eventually asked me to join them for the Pan Am Games. It was really that simple!

The Games were held in August, and conveniently that was the only month of the year that we had off from Hockey Canada. I told Allen that I would have to get clearance from Hockey Canada in order to go to Rio, so we checked with them first.

I was granted permission. Hockey Canada had a good idea about the personal issues I was facing at the time, and they were probably happy that I was getting out of the country and getting involved with something that would help keep me in shape for the sledge hockey season (I really was in pretty good shape physically at that point, as all I did besides speaking and broadcasting was workout and train for the season).

I wasn't a sitting volleyball star by any stretch of the imagination, but I did contribute with my leadership skills and because I could really serve the ball well, I was used as a serving specialist at key times in some games during the Pan Am Games.

The team was really a bit of a rag tag outfit at the time and expectations were low, but guess what? We shocked everybody by playing well enough to win a bronze medal at the Pan Am Games! I was so happy for those guys, and so happy they let me be a small part of something so special.

I was never going to stay with them for very long as I mentioned…not at my age and not with my sledge hockey commitments and speaking career taking up so much of my time. But thanks to a chance encounter at the University of Ottawa, I became a very rare two-sport medalist for Team Canada in international competition!

It was such fun and an experience I'll never forget. I told the team after the Pan Am Games I wouldn't be returning and thanked them, and made my way to our sledge hockey training camp.

Boy, did I ever get the gears from the guys when I arrived there! I was teased mercilessly about my "two sport" career and they basically had a laugh with me. I got my revenge on them in a unique way, however.

I arranged with the coaching staff for our sledge hockey team to play a little sitting volleyball in the gym as a team bonding exercise. All of the sledge hockey players got in their chairs and they soon discovered – it ain't as easy as it looks! We had a blast playing and they discovered a new respect for the sport. I was never teased about my "two sport" career by them again.

I learned a valuable lesson from all of this, and I tell this story at most of my talks as well. Great things can happen if you just put yourself out there, go out and meet a few people, and get involved in something. Just imagine – if I had driven home that night that marvelous experience with the sitting volleyball team would never have happened for me.

You never know what can happen when you just stick around and talk to someone. I am eternally grateful to Phil Allen and his team for that day at the University of Ottawa and to Soldier On for being the reason I was there in the first place.

Just goes to show you yet again – never give up.

CHAPTER 21

SLED HEAD

Also during this time period in 2007, there were a lot of cameras around our sledge hockey team. A man named David McGillivray and his crew was putting together a documentary on sledge hockey with the working title of SLED HEAD.

They started following us in September 2007, and the plan was that they'd stay with us through the world championships coming up in Boston in April, 2008. The documentary would then be released that September on CTV's W5.

I'm sure you are not surprised by the fact that I was front and center and always in front of the cameras for this project.

I was still miserable during this time period in my personal life, and if you watch the documentary it is noticeable. I am acting in it like I am King Shit but in my mind I'm just a piece of shit. I was totally separated from my family during most of the filming and when I re-watch the program, I can see that I was subconsciously trying to let the world know that I wasn't a happy person.

On the ice was a different story. Things were continuing to go well with the team. There was interest in CTV in us because we were good – we were very good. Coming on the heels of the worlds the year prior, we were getting a lot of attention and this film might really catapult us even higher on the publicity charts.

Our play merited that kind of attention. After some disappointments in previous years, things were really cooking with us, we were constantly winning tournaments, and we really expected another world title by the time the SLED HEAD crews were finished up with us in Boston.

Steve Yzerman had always been a big supporter of our program, and he called us before the tournament to wish us luck. He told us not to take anything for granted, as winning at the world level was never easy, as he certainly knew first hand. That call only boosted our already high confidence even higher.

The crowds in Boston were huge and enthusiastic. We dominated all week, including a 5-0 rout over our top rivals Norway, and we headed into the gold medal game again against Norway brimming with confidence.

However Stevie Y's words turned out to be prophetic…it never is easy to win at the world level.

Norway was ready for us this time, and we had a real fight on our hands. Billy Bridges (Sami-Jo Small's husband), gave us a 1-0 lead with his early goal, but he got tossed out of the game with 15 seconds to go in the opening period after taking a penalty, resulting in a 5-on-3 advantage for Norway.

I mentioned earlier that you usually score on a five-on-three in sledge hockey, or get scored on if it's three-on-five against you, and we got scored on. Norway tied the game 1-1 and the score stayed that way as we went into the second intermission.

Now the pressure was really on. It was the first time the world championships were played in North America and all of our family and friends are there watching. We still felt pretty good about our chances, but a tie game after two periods is a true indication that anything can happen.

We got into penalty trouble again in the third period. Norway gets another 5-on-3 and they score again, giving them a 2-1 lead with just six minutes to go in the game.

I kept the guys thinking positive during a timeout.

"We'll tie it up and get it to overtime," I told them. I was convinced we weren't going to let this chance at another gold medal slip away from us. My personal life might have been in tatters, but on the ice I was still confident we were going to win every time out. I shared my confidence with my teammates at every opportunity.

I will never forget the end of that game on April 8, 2008. Adam Dixon scored on a great individual play with 1:20 left to tie it, and with just 9.3 seconds left in regulation time, Greg Westlake – my former back-up goalie who had moved to forward thanks to my insistence! – netted the winner to give us a 3-2 victory.

We had another world championship gold medal and boy that one was sweet! The crowd went nuts. It couldn't have been a better ending for the SLED HEAD documentary either; it really was one of our defining moments as a team.

I jumped into the stands and gave my Dad the gold medal after we got presented with it. What a special moment that was for him and I to be able to share.

We were honored by many other sports teams when we got back to Canada. The Toronto Raptors, Toronto Argos, Ottawa Senators, Edmonton Oilers and Vancouver Canucks all had us out at their games for a special presentation. We were the toast of the town in a lot of towns.

I am not going to lie and say I didn't enjoy all of that attention. I did. But all of the accolades and attention still weren't paying any bills, so when we all returned to our regular lives there was also a real letdown.

I guess I was really hoping that when SLED HEAD came out, it would lead to something that might make my life easier financially, and I'd benefit from the exposure. Maybe now with this great publicity I could finally make some real money off of all of this activity.

SLED HEAD came out that fall and it was really well done, with all 84 minutes of it airing on the W5 show. But realistically, it did nothing for me or anyone on the team. It was well produced and well received, but around the same time a United States documentary on wheelchair rugby – Murder Ball – was getting most of the attention given to these kinds of projects. Our film was Canadian so by comparison, it didn't get nearly as much publicity as Murder Ball got.

I frankly admit I was disappointed by that. I had really put myself out there; I had allowed them to film me constantly and I was brutally honest throughout, but the end result was despite my baring my soul to the world for this film, I was no better off financially as a result of its release. And that was true even after winning one World Cup, one world championship, a Paralympics gold AND having SLED HEAD released.

It was just the way it was. Being a sledge hockey goalie wasn't going to lead to riches, although I did have my speaking career going well. But I really did think that maybe there would be further opportunities for me to earn some money from my playing career (endorsements or whatever), but they never materialized.

Around this time I started seeing Team Canada psychologist Shauna Taylor. I was getting more and more well-known nationally and on the surface, everybody thought I was doing great. I wasn't, so I reached out to her for help.

I was the King of Bullshit. I'd speak to a group and go home. My life during this period was lived either at an event, playing or training for sledge hockey, or in bed in my apartment.

I was doing OK financially with the speaking, but I'd spend every cent I got either gambling, or through my nose or mouth, by abusing drugs and alcohol. Everybody might have thought I was Jesus, but I felt lower than I had ever felt before.

I had my sports and my pills and my alcohol, and that was about it. I had an affair with Jack Daniels too at this time – and that affair, like most with the bottle, didn't end well.

I mention all of this to let you know something – never judge a book by its cover. In other words - never assume someone who is always smiling is happy inside. You never know what's going on in someone's life.

Here I was a motivational speaker, an Olympic, World Cup and world championship gold medal winner, in a sport I loved. And I was a mess. It was a pretty low period for me, despite my appearances.

And it was about to get even worse.

CHAPTER 22

DARKER TIMES

I have to say that from the time SLED HEAD was released up until the next Paralympics was the lousiest stretch of my life up until that point. That is saying something, but it was true.

Team Canada was still competing well during this time – that part was still going more than OK. A highlight certainly came early in 2009 at the University of British Columbia, in a four-team tournament featuring Canada, the United States, Norway and Japan. We won the final game of that event 1-0 after seven shootout rounds. I was terrific in that game.

Dave Randorf of TSN interviewed me afterwards and said some really good things about me. When the interview was over he said I had done a great job promoting the team and when my playing days were done, I should look into doing color work, and that TSN would be happy to have me. It really meant a lot to me for him to encourage me like that – especially since it was obvious my playing career was winding down. He would later on become an important part in my entering the broadcasting field, but that didn't happen for a while yet.

Although I still had maybe a couple of years of playing time left, I was getting near the end of my sledge hockey career and deep down I realized that. Being aware of that fact only made my drinking problem worse, and I was a very unpleasant person to be around during those years leading up to the 2010 Olympics in Vancouver.

I have always believed that you have to live your life without regrets and I take full responsibility for everything I've done in my life. That said, if I could go back and do just one thing differently, it would be to change the way I behaved in the year or so leading up to those Olympics.

I wasn't a very pleasant person to be around then. My ego took over. I put myself in a category that was above everyone else on my Team Canada sledge hockey team, and I regret that time very much. If I wasn't as good a goalie as I was, I would have been thrown off the team hundreds of times.

I admit it now. I was a prick.

Back then I was taking so many mind altering substances that I was a complete mess. I was very cruel to a lot of people. I never blamed the drugs for my behavior, but I became a horrible person when I was abusing as much as I did then.

I must have been taking 30-40 pills of day of some sort, including oxi. My pain killers were like skittles to me, I just wolfed them down. When I was clear headed enough to apologize to people I did, but most of the time I was an arrogant so and so that thought he was above the rules.

Nothing I can do about that time period now except to apologize again to anyone I hurt. I was truly hurting, both physically and mentally, but that's no excuse. I really do wish I could have that time back again and live it over.

I was playing tremendously well despite all of this drama I was creating. Our team was loaded with talent and we were very, very good. We entered the 2009 world championships in the Czech Republic as clear favorites, and we walked through the early stages of it.

By this time my ego is totally out of control, I am just full of myself. I put myself ahead of all my teammates and acted like I was the only guy who counted. I was in a very toxic personal relationship at this time as well, and my drug and alcohol addiction was getting extremely serious.

However on the ice, I was still managing to play at the highest level possible. Our team was unstoppable and frankly so was I. At the 2009 worlds, despite all my personal problems, nobody could score on me. And when I mean nobody, I mean nobody!

I did not give up a single goal in regulation time in the entire event. We started the tournament with four straight shutout wins, all of them in convincing fashion. And I didn't allow a regulation goal in the final two games either.

But we still lost. You read that right. I played six games at the 2009 world championships, and the only goal I allowed was in a shootout to the United States in our fifth game. We lost the game 1-0, and that loss knocked us out of the gold medal game. The one goal I did surrender wound up costing us a goal medal.

I'll never forget that one goal either. The shot went off the post, off of my back, and into the net. It was more of a fluke than anything else. We were in total dis-belief about what had happened and a few of us went out drinking after that game and just got hammered. It was not a pretty sight.

I played in the bronze medal game. I get another shutout. We beat Japan 2-0 to win the bronze medal. My stats line from the tournament – six games played, six regulation shutouts. The one goal I allowed in the shootout to the US was it, but it was enough to cost us a gold medal we should have won.

You must admit that's pretty good goaltending. I was an excellent goalie in my prime, there's no doubt about that. But I had the worst attitude in the world as a teammate, and like I said, if I wasn't as good as I was I'd have been kicked off the team.

I was still seeing the Team Canada psychologist during this time to try and deal with my issues, but I really should have been getting constant therapy and I couldn't afford that. I really struggled in the years leading up to the 2010 Games mentally.

I thought a lot about suicide once again. To the world I was Paul Rosen, star goaltender; but I knew even that would come to an end soon, no matter how well I had played in the Czech Republic. That thought combined with my drug habit sent me into a deep depression. I was nothing without hockey in my mind.

I was about to turn 49 years old. My health is starting to decline again, and my attitude was horrible. Corbin Watson was an up-and-coming young goalie who had been tabbed as my replacement, so I knew that my time on the international stage was running out.

I had a serious drug addiction and all that kept me from completely going over the edge is sledge hockey – and soon enough, that would be over for me. All that's left for me as a player is most likely the 2010 Olympics in Vancouver.

I knew before those Games started that it would be my last major event as a player. I had no idea what I was going to do after my playing days were over, and I had no idea how I could get my personal life back in order.

But I did know one thing. We had to win the gold medal at those Vancouver Games in front of the home country crowd at all costs.

We just had to.

CHAPTER 23

VANCOUVER OLYMPICS

The 2010 Winter Olympic Games were a defining moment for our country. It was an incredible experience for everyone involved and those Games showed what a great sporting country – make that a great country period – we really are.

The men's, women's and sledge hockey teams were all announced in September, 2009. The month prior we had a training camp and the hype around the camp and training periods was enormous.

In the lead-up to the official announcement of the teams, I was doing my usual promotion job for sledge hockey. I was somewhere for what seemed like every breakfast, lunch and dinner every day during that time, as we tried to take full advantage of the extra exposure the sport would be getting since the Olympics were in Canada.

It was an exciting time, but there was also a lot of pressure. Hey, this is the Olympics and it is hockey and it is IN Canada this year. There is only one color of medal that's acceptable for a Canadian hockey team to win. That pressure comes anytime you wear a Maple Leaf on your chest, but it was really pronounced when we played at home.

The pressure to win was nothing new to me of course. I wanted that gold medal badly. But I wanted it for myself, because at that point the only thing I was concerned with was setting me up financially when the Olympics were over. I wanted it for selfish reasons.

I knew this was likely going to be it for me as a player, and certainly there would be no greater stage than this one to benefit from. Paramount Pictures had approached me with some interest in doing a movie about my life if we won another gold medal, so I was pumped about that. If that happened I might finally gain some lasting financial benefit from my decade in this sport, or so I thought. I became a man obsessed with having to win in the months leading up to those Games.

I was frankly out of control. My ego was in control of me.

But as people who really understand big egos know, having a big ego didn't mean I had self-esteem. It was the opposite. Any kind of slight towards me could bring me down so fast it wasn't even funny.

I remember one incident in particular during the training camp time leading up to the Vancouver Games. Roberto Luongo of the Canucks was the men's team goalie then and obviously the toast of Vancouver. I saw him in an elevator on the way to an event one time and greeted him warmly.

"Bobby Lou!" I greeted him.

He just looked at me with the same kind of look that I remember my mother giving me when I was being a jerk as a kid. That look just made me feel so inferior, and I felt really awful after that meeting.

Was Luongo being deliberately mean to me? I can't say. It could be he was just having a bad day, or that he didn't know who I was, or maybe that's just the way he always was and the way he treated everybody. I'm not blaming him - I hear he's a really good person. But I recount that story to show just how fragile my self-esteem was; the Canadian men's hockey team goalie didn't treat me with any respect in MY mind, so that meant I was worthless in MY mind.

I mention this not to embarrass Luongo, but only to show you how fragile I was at that time, even though I went around acting like I was the king.

I sure acted like a king when I was with my own teammates. We had three goalies, and Watson was one of them. He was going to be the guy that replaced me and I knew that. But there was no damn way that was happening in these particular Olympics. Not a chance.

I made it clear to the coaching staff – I wanted my own net for the entire tournament. I became impossible to deal with. I was the veteran on this team, I was the voice of this team, and I was going to play every game in goal - and that was the end of that.

The more I drank, and the more I took drugs, the more difficult I became to deal with. I turned into the kind of person I didn't like. I really should have been thrown off the team for acting the way I did, but all I cared about was being the star, winning the gold, and getting a movie deal that I could cash in on later. I was too important to the team for them to throw me off it and I knew it.

I really caused a lot of problems. We had three games scheduled as a tune up against Korea and I didn't even bother to show up for them. They weren't important enough for me. As I've said several times before…if I hadn't been as good as I was (no goals allowed in six games at the world championships in 2009 remember), they wouldn't have put up with me.

How I managed to hang in there was really a small miracle. They made me sign a waiver after the Korean stunt I pulled that I was on probation and told me straight out, if there were any other issues until the Games started, they wouldn't hesitate to make a change.

I didn't believe they'd actually bench me, but I just had to stay on the team and I had to play in the Olympics to ensure my future. I managed to stay out of any more trouble until the Games started in March.

It was not a good time for me personally at all, but again, I make no excuses for my behavior. And much later on I took full responsibility for the way I acted in those months leading up to the Vancouver Games and apologized to everybody involved.

But right at that time, I just had to make sure I stayed on the team and did my part by being great in goal. I wasn't concerned with anyone else's feelings, just my own.

So I watched my behavior and just did my usual thing. Despite the internal problems I was still the promotional face of the team. I'd fly to Vancouver from Toronto to make a promotional appearance, do what I had to do, and take a red-eye flight back home afterwards.

I also kept training like a fiend so I would be ready physically. I was nearly 50 years old, but by Christmas of 2009 I was probably in the best physical shape I had ever been in. I was constantly on the ice or in the gym working out, and keeping my skills sharp as a goaltender.

I loved my goaltending at that point…but I hated my life.

◘ ◘ ◘

As the 2010 Olympic Games got closer, so did the end of my playing days primarily because of my age. The thought remained a bit terrifying for me, which was probably one of the reasons I was so difficult to deal with in those days.

I had a few more speaking gigs going and I managed to get COLD-FX as a personal sponsor in this period, so things weren't too bad financially. But at the back of my mind was the pressing need to finally cash in on my playing career by the time these Olympics were over. I had a drug and alcohol habit to support too after all.

We needed to win the gold medal before any new cash would start flowing in. Paramount Pictures was getting more and more interested in a movie about my life, and that could be the bonanza I had been looking for. Another gold medal would certainly bring me a lot more exposure too, and likely result in more motivational speaking deals for me. There was so much at stake for me personally in our team winning the gold.

And Team Canada was always under pressure of course. Not much had changed in that regard – gold medal or bust. But the fact that we were playing at home was expected to help us, and our team was good enough to win no matter where we were playing. Yes, I had selfish personal financial goals that I was hoping to achieve, but I was still a very good goalie playing on a very good sledge hockey team with an excellent chance to win despite all of that drama.

There was no doubt heading into those Games that I was the number one guy in goal. There was no doubt that we should be expected to win a gold medal. I was mentally in rough shape, but I was in physically great shape to play. Our entire team was ready as we headed to training camp in Trail, B.C. shortly before the Games began.

I was not a newcomer to the Olympics by then as you already know. This was my third Olympics, and we were defending gold medalists from Torino in 2006. The experiences we all had in Salt Lake City and Torino were fantastic in their own way.

But the Olympic Games in Vancouver? Oh my heavens this took the Olympic experience to another level!

Of course everyone in the country remembers what happened in the men's and women's hockey tournaments that year. Sidney Crosby's golden goal will never be forgotten, and the women won the gold medal as well in thrilling fashion.

That was amazing for Canada…but boy did it ever ramp up the pressure on us even further.

We were treated like gold throughout the tournament once the Paralympics began. Our games were all sold out and we truly had amazing support from Canada's fans throughout the tournament. People in Vancouver couldn't get enough of the Olympic and Paralympic experience in 2010.

But from the moment that Sidney scored his golden goal, the amount of pressure on us was just insane. We always felt we had to win, but my God did we ever feel it as our turn to play got closer.

The support we had was wonderful and there's nothing like playing in front of your home fans in an Olympics. But as we watched both of Canada's other hockey teams win (watching the games together as a team), we heard on the national broadcast "John Labonte, you and the sled team are next!" He basically implied we were expected to win gold too.

The look on some of the faces of our players when that was said…well now we really knew what was at stake. We knew right then we'd never experienced the kind of pressure we'd be feeling when it was out turn to represent Canada at home.

Before all of that happened, being a part of the opening ceremonies was just astounding. The place was packed, and the place went crazy as we marched into the stadium wearing our Team Canada colors. What happened next was a real disappointment that I still am bitter about a decade later, however.

In the opening ceremonies of any Olympic Games, there's a lot of hurry up and wait. You are on your feet for hours, they take a lot of time, and you are in the stadium for hours on end.

For the athletes it is a very special occasion though. You work hard all your life for this chance, so the fact that these things drag on isn't a big deal. However it was a big deal apparently to the Hockey Canada organizers.

We were told "we had to go" in no uncertain terms right in the middle of the opening ceremonies. We had a game the next day against Italy and the organizers wanted us to be well rested, but we were all furious that we weren't allowed to stay and take part in the whole event.

We were never given a full explanation as to why we had to go back to the village so quickly, only that "It's a Hockey Canada decision" and it was made to make sure we got the proper rest we needed before the tournament began.

It was still the wrong call in my mind. There's no way we weren't going to be ready to play just because we stood around in a ceremony the day before, and for all of us (especially the first time Olympians), it deprived us of a lifetime memory that we couldn't be a part of the whole thing.

This might not seem like a big deal to some of you reading, but believe me we were pissed. However so be it – it was time to play.

We were terrific in that first game. We crushed Italy 5-0, and went on to beat Sweden and our top rival Norway easily in the next two games. We were firing on all cylinders and had crazy support from the home country fans. Things were going accordingly to plan.

When you are in the heat of an Olympic tournament, sometimes you don't have a chance to really let it all soak in. That wasn't the case for me though; I knew this was more than likely my last major event of any kind as a player, and I had dreams of stardom waiting for me personally after we won the gold medal.

Therefore I was going to savor every second of this Paralympics…and I did.

But nothing in the world could have prepared me for what happened next.

▫ ▫ ▫

Our chief competitors in international competition for most of my career were Norway and the United States. So when we wound up drawing Japan in the semi-finals, we weren't overly concerned.

All we had to do was beat them and we were in the gold medal game. Just two more victories now and we'd have it all – back-to-back Olympic gold medals, the second one in front of our adoring fans. I'd have a movie made on my life and finally get some financial gain from all of these years of playing.

The crowd was rabid and cheering us on like mad. The stage was set for a Team Canada win.

Late in the second period of that semi-final game, we led the Japan 1-0. I should probably say we led "only" 1-0, because that was a lot closer score than the one we'd been expecting. Perhaps we were playing a little too tight, and perhaps the Japanese were nice and lose because they were the underdogs and didn't feel the pressure the way we did. I'm still not sure all these years later what actually happened to us on that day.

Japan scores a fluke goal late in the second period to tie the game. We were shocked. Still, we'd been in tight games before and always come through, so to a man we felt we'd just do it again here. We'd find a way to win, and go on to the gold medal game.

It remained 1-1 as the clock ran down in regulation time. With 1:40 left on the clock, we had a defensive break-down. I looked up and saw a 3-on-none break coming my way.

I couldn't stop it. Japan scores again and now leads 2-1.

Up until that point the arena had been ear-splitting loud. When that goal went in, you could hear a pin drop. The silence was deafening.

We desperately pressed to try and tie it up, but Japan scores again with just eight seconds to play into our empty net. We lose the game in shocking fashion, 3-1.

Disaster had struck.

Our gold medal dreams are shattered. It was an absolute nightmare. In front of a rabid home crowd, which included all of my family, we suffer the most embarrassing loss in my 10 years of playing goal for Team Canada.

We lost to Japan, a team we had never lost to before in a major international competition. We were crushed.

My first thought was a simple one – my life was over. I can't even describe how devastated I was after that game.

I honestly REALLY wanted to kill myself. It's a good thing my kids were in attendance…because I think the only reason I didn't kill myself was because they would have been there to see it.

◘ ◘ ◘

We had one more game to play of course. It was the Paralympics after all. There was a bronze medal game.

Like most Canadians playing hockey, bronze isn't the color of medal we are looking for. And after that devastating loss to Japan, we were emotionally flat for the final game against Norway just a few days later.

Even though it was in Canada and the fans still cheered us on, we just couldn't muster up enough effort for one more win and some kind of a medal at least. Norway scored on a penalty shot that tied the game 1-1 in the third period, then again with just 1.1 seconds remaining in regulation time, to beat us in heartbreaking fashion, 2-1.

So not only did we not win the gold, we finished in fourth place and out of the medals. The bronze medal loss also hurt, as some kind of a medal would have been something at least, but frankly after we were eliminated from winning the tournament, we were just a beaten team.

And I was a beaten man.

In my mind I felt like my life was truly over. Everything that I had worked for was now for nothing. There would be no movie offer from Paramount – a Cinderella feel good story about a fourth place finisher just didn't cut it.

I also lost a few sponsors shortly after, including COLD-FX, and I probably lost at least another $100,000 of potential income as a result of that loss to Japan.

That was bad, but what was even worse than losing the potential money was losing the gold medal as it turned out. As badly as I had wanted to financially cash in from my career, I only realized how much I wanted to win another gold medal after we lost. We all felt that we had let the country down and failed to deliver in a tournament that was basically set up for us to win.

We were defending Olympic champions. Our team was excellent. We were on home ice and wildly cheered by Canadian hockey fans. We had all the funding and support we needed to make it happen…yet it didn't happen.

I know everyone on our team felt that bitter disappointment greatly, but it was especially bitter for me because I knew the end was near for me personally. I had also been a real jerk during the months leading up to the Olympics and now I felt even worse about my behavior. Team Canada would be happy to see the last of me, even if I hadn't been 50 years old and clearly near the end of my playing time like I was.

I did cling to a longshot hope for a while that maybe – just maybe – I'd be able to stick around a bit longer as a player and get to another world championship – or something. But it didn't take long for that balloon to burst too.

Hockey Canada took its time to lick its wounds from the loss. However in September of 2010, just as the new season was about to get rolling, they called me up and made it official.

I was told they were "going to move on" from me. I actually didn't want to retire now, especially going out the way we did, but it was 100 percent taken out of my hands. I didn't even get a real chance to plead my case.

It was done in a phone call that lasted maybe five minutes. It was so painful to me it felt like it lasted five hours.

"Well Paul, we feel it is best that you retired," I was told.

"I guess I'm retiring then" was my response. And just like that, it was over. It was heartbreaking for it to all end like that, but that's just the way it was.

Let me make this crystal clear, despite the way my playing career ended – I am eternally grateful to Hockey Canada for all they have done for me over the years. They treated me like gold and it was an honor and a privilege to have worn the Team Canada colors for as long as I did.

I made things difficult on the organization with my behavior too many times, and I take full responsibility for my actions. It was a tremendous ride I had, and Hockey Canada made it all possible. I will never forget everything they did for me.

But after more than a decade, the ride was over - I was released. I would now find out what my life would be like without sledge hockey.

I was terrified to get the answer to that.

CHAPTER 24

RETIREMENT TIME

Paul Rosen was nothing without hockey. It was all I was. That's honestly the way I felt after I was released by Team Canada in September 2010.

As I said earlier I knew that the Vancouver Olympics were likely going to be it. But knowing it in your heart isn't the same as actually knowing it – I guess I was still clinging to hope that I might get one more shot at it as a player.

But the team had younger goalies in the pipeline. Corbin Watson was ready to take over. What was happening was no different from the time I replaced Pierre Pichette back in 2003, except it was now happening to me.

Despite all of the hassles I had caused, I truly loved being a sledge hockey goalie. I loved the games. We were treated very well. I loved being the team's promoter, being asked for autographs – and despite my frustrations at times, I cherished the "role" of being a hockey player and everything that came along with it.

Despite the battles I had with Hockey Canada over the years, I thought we had a pretty good relationship. After earning an Olympic gold medal, a world championship gold medal and a World Cup gold, after all of the promotion I had done to help the sport of sledge hockey come to prominence…I felt the organization still respected me despite the jerk I had turned into as my career wound down.

However that didn't stop them from having my "retirement" phone call and making it clear that my playing days were over, whether I wanted them to be or not. I couldn't blame them for that, but it still hurt.

I went on the Team Canada website and saw the announcement of my "retirement" prominently displayed. That made it official in black and white. It was tough to see it, let me tell you.

As I said, my gratitude to Hockey Canada for the way they treated me overall over the years is huge. At the end of the day, we had both been good for each other and I was as hurt as I was not because of what they did, but because of how much being a part of Hockey Canada meant to me.

It was just time for me to move on as a player. That's all.

Anyway, that meant I had big issues to face. What the hell was I going to do with my life now?

There was going to be no final "financial home run" for me at the end of my career which I had longed for. I had dedicated more than a decade of my life to playing for Team Canada and working hard to promote the sport of sledge hockey. I had a lot of great memories and lot of great stories, but I certainly didn't have much in my bank account to show for it.

For better or worse, I had dedicated so much of my life and time to the sport that I didn't really have any kind of other career. I had started doing motivational speaking and that was at least something, but other than that I really never benefited financially from my playing career despite my best efforts.

I needed money and now that my career was ended, I was left scrambling to find something to do.

I had started dating a girl around this time and how our relationship ended perfectly illustrates where my life was at. She was with me during the Olympics and when I was playing, but she soured on our relationship as soon as the Olympics ended. After I bought her a few things, she promptly dumped me that November. I guess she saw that I wasn't going to be the gravy train she probably thought I'd be.

I was still on very poor terms with my ex-wife and with my kids for the most part, since I had barely been around for them in the decade I was playing. Now that hockey had ended for me, the motivation to keep working out was gone as well, and my physical health now began to slip too.

Not to mention – I was still drinking hard. I was still using drugs to cover my pain as well. And I was now facing all of this without having the trappings and the sense of security that came from being a Team Canada athlete.

I wasn't Paul Rosen Team Canada Paralympic goalie anymore. I was just Paul Rosen and I was totally lost.

There weren't a lot of highlights for me between the years 2010-2014 as a result of all this. However there was one HUGE positive that happened – it did mark the beginning of a significant new adventure for me.

I did manage to find a way to return to hockey…via the broadcast booth.

CHAPTER 25

ROAD HOCKEY

Before I get around to telling you about how my broadcasting career unfolded, I want to tell you a pretty nice story from 2010, as I had a chance to be a part of an inaugural event that went on to become quite the annual tradition.

My playing career had just ended, so I was feeling pretty low. But my spirits did get lifted a bit when I got a call from Kevin Shea of The Princess Margaret Cancer Foundation, a terrific organization that was always looking for ways to raise funds for cancer research. Kevin is a tremendous promoter, a great writer and a good friend of mine.

The Foundation was looking for a new fundraising event, something large enough in scale that could raise a lot of money in one shot. That is not an easy thing to do by any means for any charity.

After organizing typical events like bike rides and walks and the other traditional fundraising ventures that every charity did, they decided to have a ball hockey tournament. It was a unique idea at the time and it was a great idea, because you didn't need ice and a lot of equipment to stage a ball hockey tournament.

In September, 2010 the Foundation decided to hold a publicity event at Yonge Dundas Square in downtown Toronto. This event would help introduce their concept to the media with a celebrity road hockey game. The idea was to generate some publicity so a lot of teams would sign up for the inaugural ball hockey tournament which was coming up later that year.

The game featured a team of Celebrities facing off against a Media team, so there would be lots of coverage. The Media team had people like Stephen Brunt of The Globe and Mail, James Duthie of TSN, Lance Hornby of the

Toronto Sun, Cabbie Richards of The Score and Christine Simpson of the MSG Network. Kevin managed to get a lot of very important media personalities involved.

I was asked to be on the Celebrity team. It had such names as NHL stars Curtis Joseph and Dennis Maruk, Team Canada women's players Jennifer Botterill and Tessa Bonhomme, and Olympic figure skater Kurt Browning on it, just to name a few.

It really was quite a big deal and I was flattered they asked me to take part. Legendary NHL referee Ray Scapinello was the official, and Scotty Bowman and Pierre McGuire spoke at the opening ceremonies.

The weather was really lousy that day as it poured rain for most of the time we were out there, but it was a lot of fun. We really raised a lot of awareness for the new event coming up – Road Hockey to Conquer Cancer.

It was a cool way to promote the upcoming fundraiser (way to go Kevin!). There was fencing around the perimeter of a rink and fans were lined eight people deep around it watching the game despite the rain. Kevin did the play-by-play and everyone had a blast.

The game ended in a manufactured tie, so it went to the shootout. I was in goal for the Celebrities (and I had a pretty good day making saves if I don't say so myself!), while the Toronto Maple Leafs mascot Carlton the Bear tended goal for the Media team. Surprisingly Carlton turned out to be a pretty good goaltender!

After seven rounds of the shootout the game was still tied. Carlton let it be known that he wanted to take his shot, especially since none of the Media guys had managed to score on me! So Carlton stumbles down towards me and fires a pretty good shot that I managed to save.

Well I certainly wasn't going to be upstaged by a stuffed bear mascot! I then told the organizers that it was my turn to take a shot. They were stunned – how was I going to be able to do that, I only had one leg after all, they must have wondered.

Well if Carlton could lumber down the rink and manage to take a shot, I could certainly do the same. I took off my prosthetic leg, grabbed a forward's stick, and drenched from the rain, hopped the length of the rink and fired a rocket shot into the top right hand corner over Carlton's shoulder!

For the first time since I was a youngster, I scored the game-winning goal in a game instead of saving it! My goal gave the Celebrities the win and the fans went crazy. I got mobbed by my teammates AND by my opponents for my one-legged hop down the floor. I actually got a great shot off too for a guy shooting on one leg!

What a fun moment that was. I was treated like a hero that day at the official launch of Road Hockey to Conquer Cancer. It was terrific of Kevin to have invited me and I was so glad I could provide some light on a rainy day for everyone. It was certainly a true highlight for me during a year that was as gloomy for me personally as the weather was on that afternoon.

The event went on to become a staple over the years. Unfortunately like many other events the novel coronavirus forced its cancellation in 2020 and 2021, but Road Hockey to Conquer Cancer has raised an astounding $23 million for cancer research at the Princess Margaret Hospital Cancer Centre since its inception.

And the event all began with a Celebrity/Media exhibition game that gave me one of the most joyful moments of my life. Here's hoping this fantastic event has many more years of success, and can return with big crowds on hand again soon.

CHAPTER 26

BROADCASTING DEBUT

So I suppose it was just a natural fit for a guy like me to become a broadcaster. I was a big talker, I had been promoting sledge hockey for years, and of course I was now a former player.

Dave Randorf, who was with TSN, really helped me get started as I talked about earlier in the book. In late 2009, I did a demo for TSN and I guess I impressed them enough for them to offer me some work doing color commentary for the major sledge hockey events that were being broadcast.

Now that I wasn't an active player anymore, I was always available. And although I didn't have any technical experience, I did have a passion and knowledge for the game that I could talk about. I was delighted to get the opportunity.

I absolutely loved it right from the start. However until I got to do my first game I never realized how difficult it was going to be. This was a whole other level up than just doing some motivational talks or just being interviewed myself when I was playing. This was real work.

My first assignment was the 2011 World Cup with Vic Rauter in London. The US wound up playing Norway in the gold medal game and it was a great experience to be able to work with a real pro like that throughout that event. I got a lot of positive reviews for the job I did.

As the years went on I got work a fair amount with TSN and CBC, and eventually broadcasting work became a focal point for me. The money was good, I was treated extremely well and most importantly, it kept me involved in hockey and that was the best part of all.

I can't thank Dave enough for encouraging me, first while I was playing and then later on, to pursue broadcasting. I can't thank TSN enough for the faith they showed me in the early days. It was literally life-saving for me to be able to get a chance to work with them and find something I truly loved to do after my retirement as a player.

I'll talk a lot more about broadcasting later in the book, but let me just say that although becoming a broadcaster was a great development for me, it certainly didn't solve my financial worries. The gigs I got did pay very well, but there weren't enough of them for a full-time income. It was basically every four years with CBC for the Olympics, and annual events with TSN, or the odd special event (like the Invictus Games were in 2017, which were held at the Mattamy Athletic Centre, the old Maple Leaf Gardens. That one was especially fun to do).

My broadcasting start was a highlight of the years just after the 2010 Games ended, but there still weren't many highlights for me in my personal life unfortunately.

My marriage was over. All I could still afford was the small apartment I had in downtown Toronto, living there alone. I was away from everybody, and that was both a good and bad thing.

It was a good thing because I was a very unpleasant person to be around, so I saved my family and the few friends I had a lot of grief. It was a bad thing because not being accountable to anybody or anything (except for my broadcasting and speaking work), just made me drink more and use drugs more. It was not a pretty scene.

Those years were tough and most days were the same, unless I happened to be working. Once again the world knew me as a hockey guy, thanks to my work with TSN and later CBC, and as a motivational speaker that helped other people. But the real Paul Rosen wasn't much of anything in the years right after my playing career ended.

I did just enough to survive. I worked just enough to pay my rent, pay my bills and support my drug and alcohol habit. That was my life pretty much in a nutshell.

I would do a speaking event, getting myself all fired up to do a great talk. As soon as it was done I went home to my lonely apartment and drank Jack Daniels and popped pills.

The motivational talks I gave were very well received. After I gave a presentation to a school or a community group or a business, I was always applauded and thanked. I met a lot of great people. And I was told by many that I had really helped them deal with their issues.

I believed them…but I just couldn't seem to deal with my own issues.

There was the Paul Rosen who hid under his covers at home, afraid of the world with an estranged family and a drug habit…and then there was the Paul Rosen who was a great speaker, a guy who could fool people into thinking he was an expert on everything, and who people thought was living this wonderful life.

I must have thought about killing myself 100 times between the end of 2010 and 2014. What stopped me? To this day I wonder about that, but probably the biggest reason was that in my way of thinking, I couldn't kill myself after giving a motivational talk to children to stop them from killing themselves. I was living a lie and hated myself at that time, but I loved the people I was helping. What would happen to them if they saw that I had given up on life? It was really that thought that kept me going and kept me sane.

I was in a lot of different romantic relationships over those years as well. I destroyed every one of them. Deep down I didn't think I deserved the love of anybody, and I was convinced those relationships weren't going to work out. So I subconsciously did things to make sure they wouldn't.

When I would go to a family event the odd time to see my family, it was always with a different girl. I think I brought seven different girls to seven different events over the period of a few years. It was embarrassing to them and to me.

I was basically sabotaging my own life. I felt deep down that I wasn't deserving of happiness or love during those years, and I did everything to drive people away from me, whether they be family members or potential romantic partners.

For that four year period I thought very little of myself. Meanwhile, as I would find out in 2013, the world saw my life in a very different light.

CHAPTER 27

JUBILEE MEDAL

It's 2013 and my personal situation is still not good. I am still living alone in a small apartment, my drug problem had worsened, and I was not in close contact with any family members. I was basically withdrawing from life as the drugs were starting to take an iron grip on me, and I had no self-esteem whatsoever. My physical health was in serious decline as well. I felt like a total failure.

But that year I received a tremendous honor. As part of the Queen Elizabeth Jubilee celebrations, Canadians from all walks of life were given an award to commemorate their public service thanking them for their contribution to Canadian life.

The award was given to just 60,000 people in our country of more than 37 million people. I was one of those honored.

The award is given to "honor significant contributions and achievements by Canadians." The committee had determined that my time as a player for Team Canada and my efforts at motivational speaking entitled me to get one of these medals.

It was humbling, and I was very grateful. The award came from the government in Ottawa, and a special reception was held at Queen's Park later in the year so we could receive our medals in person.

I wasn't feeling very well at all the night of the event, but there was no way I wasn't going to go. You could only invite a few guests, so I brought my mother, my father and brother with me to the ceremony.

Talk about feeling out of place! Here I am with people like Toronto Argonauts owner David Cynamon, Robert Herjavec of Dragon's Den fame and Frank Lango, getting an award from the Prime Minister of Canada and the Governor General of Canada.

All I can think about while standing around with these people is that they are all multi-billionaires – except me! I'm standing off to the side, feeling uncomfortable, but nevertheless proud to have been given this award.

It was really a special honor. The medal cannot be worn in public, it's only to be brought out at government functions, and very few people were getting one. My self-esteem was very low at that time of my life, but I have to admit I was feeling pretty good about being included in company like that.

I was standing off to the side of the crowd, trying to be inconspicuous, when Prime Minister Stephen Harper and Governor General David Onley (who was handicapped himself) both approach us.

What a special moment. The Prime Minister taking the time to congratulate me and thank me for helping people with my motivational speaking and for what I have done for Canada. I couldn't believe it!

I also couldn't believe what my mother did then.

Prime Minister Harper turned to my father and shook his hand. "We are honored to be here" my Dad says with a smile. Then he turns to my mother.

"Can I ask you a question?" my Mom says to the Prime Minister of Canada. "Why are you giving this to my son?"

My face turns red in shame. I was so embarrassed. I went from feeling like King Shit to a piece of shit in the five seconds it took her to ask that.

Mr. Harper was so gracious and diplomatic towards her though.

"Your son is a Canadian hero," the Prime Minister told my mother. "It's what he does off the ice, as much as he did on the ice, that this medal is for."

Thank God the Prime Minister had my back at least.

I loved my Mom. But I didn't talk to her for a good seven months after that night…and the only reason I made up with her eventually is that my Dad begged me to. My God what she said hurt me so much.

That incident really summarizes the story of what my life was like at that point I guess. No matter what great things were happening to me, there was always a dark cloud around somewhere – either one that I created, or someone else did - that spoiled even the best moments. Deep down my Mom didn't think I deserved a great honor like this. And deep down I guess I didn't either, which is why I felt so hurt by her comments to the PM.

Instead of looking back at that night in pride, the memory of that evening and how my Mom acted still haunts me to this day. We wound up driving home in stony silence and what should have been a bright night turned into a dark one for me.

My Mom and I later put this incident behind us, but it was another example of how appearances can be deceiving. Other people who were there that night probably looked at us and saw a happy family celebrating a happy event. That sure wasn't us.

You never know what's really going on in anyone's life behind the scenes friends. This just serves as another reminder to always be kind. Smiles can be deceiving.

CHAPTER 28

ANOTHER OLYMPICS

So between my retirement in 2010 as a player and 2014, my life consisted primarily of giving motivational talks to others while trying not to kill myself. I was a walking and talking contradiction.

My body is starting to break down a little more, I'm seriously addicted to drugs and I am missing being a Team Canada athlete like you couldn't possibly imagine. Getting to do some work on broadcasts with TSN was great, but those were only short gigs and I wound up missing being a player even more once they were completed. Broadcasting the games just made me realize what I was missing by not being on the ice any more.

The irony was…all I did was complain during the last 18 months of my playing career, but now I longed for those days once again. I missed the actual playing. I missed being a member of a team. I missed the travel. And I really missed being a part of the Olympics more than anything.

But thanks to my broadcasting career, there was one big bright spot. I was going to get a chance to go to another Olympics.

◘ ◘ ◘

The early years of the 2010s marked the start of my broadcasting work with TSN. Thank God for that, as it gave me something to do for a bit of time that I truly did love almost as much as playing.

I had worked for TSN for about five events when in late 2013, I was approached by CBC about doing color commentary for the upcoming 2014 Paralympics in Sochi, Russia.

I was very excited to have that opportunity. I wound up working with Rob Snoek, a terrific person and a terrific broadcaster. We didn't get to travel to Russia for the Paralympics, but we did broadcast the games from a studio at the CBC building just down the street from where I was living at the time.

We wound up doing a total of six Canadian games, which was really a great experience. It would have been so much better to have actually been there of course, but this was the next best thing.

But talk about the difference of doing play-by-play off a monitor, instead of being there! Not being there in person made it that much tougher to do the job well. I don't know how Rob was able to be so good at play-by-play the entire week, but he was.

I loved the work and really embraced the challenge. I would be at the job night and day, and by that I mean all night and all day, because of the time difference. I would get into the studio at 3 am, sometimes earlier, and we would broadcast the games while watching them on the TVs we had set up in a special room.

During one of the games, we lost the satellite feed that was coming into our monitor. I was able to see another TV that hadn't lost its feed that Rob couldn't see from where he was positioned, so I actually did a little play-by-play before the satellite came back. Now I know how tough that part of the job is first hand!

I always went the extra mile in preparing to be on air. I would go in well before I had to be there and sometimes stay overnight just watching tapes of previous games, so I'd be up to speed on everything. Scott Moore, executive producer of the broadcasts, would see me in there sometimes putting in the extra time, and he and others were very impressed with my work ethic.

But to me it was more than just work; it was a salvation from the life I was living when I wasn't kept busy doing things like this that I just loved. I was well paid, but I certainly gave them more than their money's worth.

Truth is I really didn't even want to come back home after those games were over.

Team Canada met the United States in the semi-final that year. Sledge hockey was broadcast mostly on the CBC's cable stations and online, but if they had made it to the gold medal game, that game would have been broadcast on CBC throughout the country.

NEVER GIVE UP

We were hoping Canada would get there as that would have been great exposure for both Rob and I, but it wasn't to be. The Americans beat Canada 3-0, so there went another great possible opportunity for me. A chance at some national exposure certainly wouldn't have hurt my chances at getting some more work down the road.

I was anything BUT a homer broadcaster. Being recently removed from playing didn't stop me from calling it like it was. Canada could have, and should have, done better and I let people know it.

Corbin Watson was good in goal throughout the tournament but he could have been better in that game against the US. Afterwards he apologized for his and the teams' performance, but I said right on air "He doesn't have to apologize, he has to play better."

I'm sure Hockey Canada wasn't all that thrilled with some of the things I said, but like I said, I called it the way I saw it. That's what they were paying me to do.

That whole experience was amazing. I couldn't wait to get into work every day. As the Olympics wound down, I started counting down the days – but not in anticipation, in dread of the Games being over.

Three more days, I thought...then two more days...and finally the last day. Just like that it was over and done with.

I was well paid for just five days of work and it was terrific. But the moment the job ended, my usual life resumed. It went right back to being the same thing for me right after the Paralympics ended. My hermit lifestyle resumed.

I spent that money pretty quickly on drugs, and what was left over went to rent and essentials. I immediately returned to a life where I was just trying to survive, to stay financially afloat, as I slipped deeper and deeper into alcohol and drug usage. I continued basically ignoring my family and friends for a lot of those years too.

Once again I was back on my miserable treadmill. And once again, to the rest of the world I was Paul Rosen, TV analyst and motivational speaker, a guy who had his act together.

But my act was never together. If the world had seen how miserable I was most of the time from 2010-2014, they never would have believed it.

Once the Olympics were done, so was I.

CHAPTER 29

DOWNWARD SPIRAL

My "just trying to survive" lifestyle continued for the next few years. However at the same time, my motivational speaking career was continuing along pretty well.

How ironic eh? I was the motivational speaker who couldn't seem to motivate himself.

I was doing a fair number of talks to schools, community groups and businesses. I had even started getting a few gigs from Hockey Canada, as we'd put the past behind us and moved on from my playing days. I never thought I'd be getting any work from them, but I did.

My goalie coach Jamie McGuire was very helpful during this time period. He arranged for me to talk to several hockey teams about the importance of dedication and hard work to their success. That was right up my alley because despite all the difficulties I was experiencing, I was always a hard worker at everything I did.

I prepared for my broadcasts the same way I prepared for games when I was a player. I spent countless hours working on the craft and it did pay off for me. Giving a message like that to young hockey players was something I certainly could do with full credibility.

My motivational speaking opportunities continued and although I basically went off the cuff in most of them, I spoke from the heart too. A lot of people were still approaching me and telling me how much the talk I gave meant to them. That certainly counted for something.

I had steady annual work with TSN right from the end of the Sochi Olympics in 2014 to 2018, and I did other events besides the Paralympics for CBC like the World Cup and World Cup Challenge, and other sledge hockey events.

My work was always well received and I enjoyed it, I won't lie about that. There just wasn't enough of it to provide me with anything more than a meager living, however.

When I was speaking, or when I was broadcasting, it was really this simple – when the light went on, Paul Rosen came on. I came alive. I put aside my own miserable life and concentrated on doing what I could to either create a great broadcast, or help other people with the message I was delivering.

As soon as the light went off, or the talk ended, Paul Rosen just went home to vegetate and do his drugs. I felt like a nothing when I had nothing to do.

Unfortunately for me, there were far too many times that I had nothing to do.

◘ ◘ ◘

One thing that hadn't changed for me on a positive note was that I still had the Paralympics to look forward to every four years, and that truly was a Godsend.

It looked like I was even going to get to travel to South Korea for the 2018 Paralympics. CBC hired me back to do the color again and told me I'd likely be able to travel there to do the games live this time. I was really pumped by the thought that I would get a chance to be there in person.

Finances came into play once again however, as CBC decided at the last minute it wasn't financially prudent to send a crew to broadcast the Paralympics, especially after spending so much money on the Olympic Games themselves. I was disappointed, but I knew that I could be as bitter as I wanted, it wasn't going to help. And at least I still had the gig to do the games off of the monitor again at the CBC building on Front Street.

2018 was turning out to be a pretty good year on the broadcasting front for me. In the months prior to the Olympics I had done some more stuff for Hockey Canada a few times. The Mattamy Athletic Centre was being used more and more for para ice hockey and I also got to do some events there. Often I was asked to give some pep talks to the players afterwards as well.

I loved being at the old Maple Leaf Gardens. It is still a hockey mecca to me. Ryerson University did a wonderful job creating a mini-version of the actual old arena inside such a marvelous building. It also contains a great gym and fitness center.

I got over the disappointment of not being able to go do the 2018 Paralympics in person pretty quickly. I started making the same trek back and forth from my apartment to the CBC studios that I had made in 2014, and just taking that walk with somewhere important to go to always put a spring in my step.

I felt really good for a while. My self-worth was as high as it had been in a long time, and I always felt thankful going into the studio (and once again, I worked far longer hours than they were paying me for).

It was like I was living another life when I was broadcasting. Whenever I had the opportunity to do something that I really enjoyed, I just came alive. Walking towards the CBC studio every day was terrific, as I felt I was needed and I was in a role that I was good at.

For as long as the Paralympics lasted, my mood would be elevated and I'd forget about how I was usually living my life. The trouble for me was that the Games didn't last very long.

It was an excellent tournament that year and Team Canada had a real crack at the gold medal game. Canada went through the early stages just sailing along in fact.

Dominic Larocque was playing goal for Canada now. He had lost a leg in the war in Afghanistan, so his was a compelling story to talk about. He was terrific in net and Canada made it to the gold medal game against the United States.

Canada carried a 1-0 lead deep into the third period of that game. The US pulled its goalie and Rob Armstrong missed an open net that would have sealed the win. The Americans wound up tying the game with just 42 seconds left, sending it into overtime.

The US was playing on emotion. Their coach, Jeff Sauer, was diagnosed with pancreatic cancer before the Olympics and had passed away before the Games began. With that as a source of motivation, they were not going to be denied in this one.

Brody Roybal, their top player, and the other superstars they had on that roster, were too much for Canada to handle during the four-on-four overtime. They dominated scoring just 20 seconds into the extra period, giving the US a 2-1 win. It really was an inspiring story to bring to the viewers.

Canada won the silver medal. We all know how Canadians feel about medals that aren't gold in color, but it was a great Games none the less.

The entire tournament was an awesome rush for me emotionally. I loved working every moment of it. But as soon as it ended, I headed back to my tiny apartment and back to my lonely life. That's where the trouble really began.

My last walk home after the tournament was over was really depressing. I was limping a bit as my left hip was bothering me a lot. Since 2016 I had been told that at some point I would need hip replacement surgery, but I had put it off. I wouldn't be able to do that for much longer.

All of my years of playing in goal, combined with walking with an artificial right leg, had caused my left hip to degenerate badly. When I was busy doing broadcasts or doing my talks, I was able to ignore the pain most of the time and when I wasn't, I resorted to the drug usage, the pain killers and the alcohol, to help mask the pain.

After the 2018 Paralympics ended I could barely walk, it was getting that bad. I knew after those Games that I would have to have the surgery. That thought alone only added to my depression.

I had a few more speaking gigs later that year, along with doing the World Cup for TV and the Canadian Tire Challenge in Bridgewater, Nova Scotia. The rest of the time I just sat around moping, and really started feeling the pain in my hip.

I was in pure agony by the time the CTC was over. I returned home from that event and knew that I just couldn't put it off any longer, so I underwent hip replacement surgery on December 13, 2018.

One of the reasons I had put it off was that I just couldn't figure out how I was going to recuperate from a surgery like that at my age, especially with the drug habit I had. That kind of surgery had come a long way and I was told by many people having it done that it was well worth the rehab time, but I spent about two years dreading it and the work I would have to do during my rehabilitation.

But there was just no choice left; the pain was too severe so I had the operation. It was a success, and I was in the hospital for 10 days.

While I sat in that hospital bed, I had nothing else to do but lie there and think. That was definitely not something I needed while being in the mental shape I was in.

I was in severe pain. I had a long road ahead to recovery. I was addicted to drugs and pain killers. And I was in a deep and severe depression.

NEVER GIVE UP

Just before I was released to go home from the hospital to my tiny apartment, the seeds were planted in my mind.

Many, many times over the years I had thought about the possibility of killing myself. This time I was going to do it.

CHAPTER 30

FATEFUL NIGHT

It was quiet in my tiny apartment the night of January 30, 2019. The TV was still on, the volume turned low. My artificial leg was leaning against the wall.

I had left my keys and my health card on a table near the door for whoever found me, so they would know who I was, along with the suicide notes I had written for my family.

I pulled the blankets over my head and closed my eyes. I was sure I had taken more than enough pills to kill me, and I just waited for the end to come. Finally it would be over I thought. Finally I would have some peace.

The end did not come.

After lying there for a while, I began to panic. Why weren't these pills doing anything? I had taken 35 of them for Christ sake!

I stumbled out of bed and although my recollections of what happened next are foggy for good reason, I must have ingested some kind of poison from my kitchen cleaning supplies in a desperate attempt to finish the job. I later was told I had swallowed a whole bottle of Windex.

I got back into bed, basically delirious by now, and again closed my eyes praying I would soon be out of my misery.

It was then that I felt a burning sensation in my stomach. It got worse and worse. It felt like my stomach was on fire. It became unbearable, and the pain I had was just insane. I honestly thought pieces of my insides were on fire.

I became violently ill. I must have vomited for a good half hour, really feeling that I was going to barf my internal organs right up there on the floor. As drugged up as I was with all those pills, they didn't mask the incredible pain I felt. It was excruciating.

The pills hadn't killed me. I was just a total mess lying there on the floor in my vomit, laughing and crying at the same time at my ineptitude. I couldn't even kill myself properly.

Shaking, barely able to stand, I managed to call 911 for help. I slumped to the floor, crying from the agony, hoping that maybe I would be dead before anybody arrived.

❏ ❏ ❏

What exactly happened after that will always be a bit of a blur to me, as I was in very bad shape.

I do remember the police arriving, and I remember that they were very kind to me. They talked to me, found out what I had done, and were very helpful and compassionate towards me. The paramedics arrived shortly after and took me to the emergency wing of St. Michael's Hospital in Toronto.

I wasn't in any shape to protest or try and do any further damage to myself. I had called 911 because the pain was just too much to bear and when I realized I wasn't going to die, that I was just going to suffer, I needed someone to help me. I had vomited out all the pills after all.

The doctors at St. Mike's examined me and I was immediately admitted into the emergency psychiatric ward of the hospital. They put me on saboxone, a drug that is mainly used to wean people off of opiate, and gave me 18 milligrams of it to start. After they had stabilized me and had me placed in a hospital bed, I was committed to undergo psychiatric evaluation for 72 hours.

The doctor who treated me said I could voluntarily agree to be placed in their psychiatric program or refuse to be, but either way I was not leaving the hospital until I was properly evaluated.

I was defeated. It is hard to explain even now, several years later, what exactly was going through my mind after I had attempted to kill myself. I guess the biggest thing I felt was a sense of resignation. I had thought of trying to kill myself hundreds of times over the years and I finally had made the attempt – and I had failed at it.

Now that I was still alive, I wasn't thinking of trying to do it again. I wasn't thinking of doing anything. I was just too tired, and wanted to sleep and not have to deal with what I had done.

I agreed to be committed for the psychiatric evaluation. I guess I wanted to find out why I had sank low enough to do this horrible thing; I had tried to end my life - and scar my family - by killing myself.

Speaking of my family, one of my clearest memories of those first few hours after being found was the look of disappointment in the faces of my daughters when they arrived at the hospital and found out the details. They seemed to be unable to comprehend why I had done what I had done.

I can't blame them, because I really didn't understand it either. Why now, after thinking about it for so long, did I finally break down and do something like this? I guess needing to know the answer to that was why I co-operated with the doctors at the hospital the way I did.

If I wanted to find some answers as to why I tried to kill myself, I needed to live. That's sounds a bit ridiculous I know, but it is the best way I can describe my inner thoughts in those first few hours.

My daughters were crushed. 48 hours before my suicide attempt, they had attempted to FaceTime me but had failed. I had talked to them on the phone the day I tried to commit suicide, but I never told them my plans. They simply couldn't come to grips with what I had done.

Nikki was especially hurt. She realized that I had been living a lie, that I was keeping my misery inside of me while I was giving motivational talks to others, telling them to never give up.

Our relationship still hasn't recovered as I write this; it's my ardent hope that one day she can forgive me for deceiving her and the world the way I did.

I had sunk as low as you can go in life, sunk so far down that I had tried to end my life. By the grace of God I hadn't, so now I had to try and learn something from this and find a way to move on.

I was kept under observation at St. Michael's Hospital for three days. On February 2, 2019, I was committed to the psychiatric ward of Toronto General Hospital.

I was there for 17 days. I was looking for some answers but before I found them for myself, I discovered just how over-burdened our health care system really is.

CHAPTER 31

GETTING CARE

The health care professionals in our society are saints. They really are.

They have to deal with so many issues, so many people who need help, and as the years go by they have to do it with fewer and fewer resources due to government cutbacks and an aging population.

So many people need help. And during this time of my life, I was certainly one of them.

It didn't take me long to see firsthand how challenging it is for these health care professionals. I was supposed to be taken by ambulance from St. Michael's Hospital to Toronto General Hospital due to the fact that I had just attempted suicide; I was supposed to have been be watched carefully in the first few days afterwards, which is why they had admitted me to a psych ward.

However there was just too much demand on their services when I was ready to be moved, so my daughter Stephanie had to take me in a cab (with no medical people helping her), to Toronto General Hospital by herself.

That was just the beginning.

When I arrived at Toronto General and was admitted, there was an overflow of patients in the ward. There were people with every kind of psychiatric case you can imagine in that ward, and all in the same area no matter how severe the patient's problems were.

Some people had only mild depression. There were people like me who had tried to kill themselves. There were people who were very dangerous to themselves and everybody around them. It was quite a mix.

One guy in particular was completely off the rails. He was psychotic and I later found out he was finding a way to avoid his meds on a regular basis, so he became wildly unpredictable.

I was put on the same floor as this man once they processed my paperwork. About five or six days into my stay, one night this guy somehow got out of the restraints they'd put him in when he became unmanageable (which was a lot of the time apparently). He clearly needed to be isolated from other people, but due to the financial issues our system is facing, he and I were put on the same floor.

At around 3 am on this night I woke up to find him standing over my bed, threatening to kill me! It was absolutely terrifying and fortunately I was able to call someone to help get him under control.

For the next three days, I didn't leave my room. If the whole point of this was for me to get better mentally, things weren't off to a very good start with that kind of floor mate.

But no matter the challenges, I had decided that I did want to get better. I came to realize that I was sick.

I really wanted to find out why I was acting the way I was, why I so often felt the way that I did, and why I had tried to end my life. My depression had been chronic throughout my life as you have just read, and it was time for me to discover why and time for me to get better mentally.

The people in my life who found out about my attempted suicide were floored. Most of them had thought, he's Paul Rosen, a guy with so much going for him, and he does something like this? How could he?

They wanted to know the answer to that question. So did I.

I did recover physically from the trauma I did to myself on January 30 while I was in the hospital, and the staff looked after me the best they could. I was heavily sedated a lot of the time from the anti-depressant drugs they gave me, but I did improve in a lot of ways thanks to the care I received (despite having to deal with a psycho early on!).

One of the reasons they kept me for as long as they did is that my daughters had to go and clear out my apartment, as the plan was that I was going to move in with Stephanie so I would have someone around me at all times. While they were cleaning my apartment out, they found the letters I had written to them, my suicide notes. The pain they both experienced from that was enormous, and it only made me feel worse about what I had done to them by trying to end my life.

Near the end of my time at Toronto General, I was assigned a therapist who would be working with me when I was released, along with a doctor.

Her name was Eva and she was a tremendous help to me right from the start. I met her for the first time on February 17, 2019 at Addiction Services York Region (ASYR), and it was then that I really began my road to recovery.

Two days after that first meeting, I was discharged. I moved in with my daughter Stephanie and her husband Eric. It was a full house, as they had two kids, and my other daughter Nikki was also living there with her boyfriend Justin.

I was just thankful to be alive, and thankful I had family that I could move in with. When I saw how stressed our health care system is, it may me feel sorry for anyone who had to depend on it for longer periods and for those who were totally alone with no family to help them. What would happen to them? It was a sad thought.

I was a lucky man in so many ways. Now I had to find a way to truly believe it.

■ ■ ■

Throughout February and March, all I thought about was getting better. My family really helped me and I am very grateful for them. Living with them made all the difference.

I didn't do very much of anything for those two months, I just concentrated on healing myself mentally. I'd have breakfast, take a walk, and just allow myself the time I needed to understand why I had done what I had done.

I went through just about every emotion possible during this time. I still felt depressed a lot for sure; I also felt deep shame at what I had put my family through by what I had done. But I also began to see that I was responsible for the way I was feeling, not anyone else.

The world saw me as someone who had a lot going for him. The world was right. I just didn't (or maybe couldn't) see myself the same way the world saw me.

I had come to finally understand how I had sabotaged my life over and over again. I had failed to live my life the way I told other people to live their lives. I needed to take my own advice and allow myself to be happy. It was a choice I could make, even when circumstances were bleak.

Those weren't easy days, I won't lie about that. I was heavily medicated on prescribed anti-depressants, as most people who attempted suicide were.

However I was seeing a therapist, which really helped me uncover the answers I was looking for.

I embraced the therapy sessions fully. I got into every program they offered, and I dove into as many things as possible to stay mentally active and be involved with people.

On February 19, I had my first appointment with Kevin Keroac, who became my addiction counselor. There were a lot of reasons why I had done the unthinkable and attempted suicide, but the biggest reason was this - my addiction to narcotics and alcohol. I had to stop abusing my body with those substances, that's all there was to it. The key to my long-term mental health would be getting clean and sober and staying that way.

There are a lot of steps you have to take on your road to recovering your mental health I found out, but the most important one is to acknowledge you need help in dealing with your addictions.

Those pills I took on the night of January 30, 2019 were the last ones I put into my body. As I write this book more than two and a half years later, I have not touched another narcotic or had a sip of alcohol.

Kevin was a tremendous source of strength and support for me. Brent Sopel, the former Chicago Blackhawks player, was another wonderful person I got to know who helped me a great deal during this time period and remains a friend. For all the bad that there is in the world, you can have faith that there is more good than bad when you see people like that care about your well-being so much.

I had to take anti-depressant medication daily for three months after my suicide attempt. I was slowly weaned off of it. I made a vow to my family and friends – and most importantly to myself – that I would never head down the road I went down again. I vowed to stay clean and sober.

It is a vow I will keep for as long as I live.

◘ ◘ ◘

Thanks to people like Kevin and Brent, and thanks mostly to my family, I began to recover. Physically I had never felt better, as I was walking all the time and not abusing any substances. My mind was slowly clearing out of the drug-infused fog it had been in for years.

One of the biggest challenges that recovering abusers have to face is to understand how badly their abuse is affecting them. Here's another great irony; the only real way to see how much drugs are affecting you is to stop using them.

However unless you stop, you often go on thinking that the drugs and alcohol have nothing to do with the problems you are facing. The fact is – your problems are being largely caused by the drugs and alcohol. My problems certainly were.

As you have read throughout this book, even when things were going well for me, I found ways to sabotage my happiness. My miserable behavior came largely from my dependence on drugs and alcohol. I just couldn't see it. I was too far gone.

The moment I became clean was the moment I saw the world clearly for the first time in decades. I had to hit absolute rock bottom to see up I suppose. That was a bitter lesson to learn, but I learned it during those three months of rehabilitation I went through – rehabilitation on both my mind and body.

I had been given a second chance to live and live properly. I was going to take it. By the grace of God I had been spared.

By late March I was well into my recovery. As I got better I began to wonder what I was going to do now to support myself. My family had saved me by taking me in, but what was the future going to hold for me? I was turning 59 years old in a month…and I now had to find a way to restart my life and make a living again.

I had been in this predicament throughout my life as you have read. But this time felt different – I somehow knew deep down that the rest of my life would be the best of my life. I would live more authentically and live clean and sober, and the rest would take care of itself.

But what could I do? Would I still have any credibility as a motivational speaker after what had happened? Would I ever be able to do any broadcasting after what had happened? Was there something else out there for me to do for a living perhaps?

On March 26, 2019, I received a phone call that started answering those questions for me.

CHAPTER 32

BROADCASTING AGAIN

I had always been an outsider among the people that ran both Hockey Canada and the International Paralympic Committee.

I've documented my tussles with Hockey Canada in this book, but my relationship with the International Paralympic Committee (IPC) was also pretty rocky. A lot of my Hockey Canada conflicts stemmed from my brash speaking style and the arrogant way I acted on the team, but with the IPC it was always about the way I played on the ice.

Even though I was a goalie, I played a physical style out there. I didn't let any player get near my goal and I was never hesitant to get in anyone's face when the going got rough. That's just the way I was whenever I was on the ice.

I say I played physical. They say I played dirty.

Maybe that wasn't the only reason I never did anything for the IPC, but it must have played a part. It was only natural that a crazy promoter like me and the governing body of the sport would try and work together; while I was constantly out there being the voice of Team Canada's sledge hockey team, I was also promoting the overall sport of sledge hockey and the Paralympics.

I had become a broadcaster after retiring as you know, and I was always available to the IPC if they had wanted someone to help them with any of their broadcast productions (which they did a lot of on their own), or someone to help spread the message about Paralympic athletics by using my speaking abilities. However there was nothing ever offered to me – until that March phone call came, just two months after my attempted suicide.

I have to admit that I was totally shocked when Sacha Beck of the IPC called me up right out of the blue.

"We want you to work with us," he told me. And the work that they wanted me to do with them was pretty sweet.

The sledge hockey world championships were about a month away in the Czech Republic. The IPC was doing its own broadcast of the event and they wanted me to be the color person for all 20 games of the tournament, which would take place over seven days.

It was an incredibly challenging assignment to be doing that many games, but the thought of getting back to doing something I loved tugged at my heart strings. Also, having this chance to finally work for the IPC directly might lead to more work in the years to come.

They wanted me to leave for the Czech Republic on April 23, and they needed an answer soon. However my first thought was…am I even going to be allowed to go by my doctors? And my second thought was…should I be doing this so soon after I tried to kill myself?

I'll be honest; I wanted to do it almost right from the moment I was asked. But I knew that it was very possible I wouldn't be allowed to travel, especially overseas and alone to do work, so soon after my suicide attempt.

The rehab was going well. I was involved in every program they had. I had been clean and sober for the past two months and was feeling pretty good. However I was just two months removed from the suicide attempt, I was still taking subscribed daily anti-depressant medication, and I had to check in with my therapist on a regular basis.

I thanked the IPC for the offer and said I would get back to them as soon as I could. I didn't tell them anything about my suicide attempt or my drug addiction. At that point only my family and a very few select other people knew what had happened to me. If the IPC had known, I'm sure they would never have asked me in a million years.

I went to see Dr. Keroic. I fully expected him to say that I shouldn't go. His response was the exact opposite of what I was thinking he might say.

"This will be amazing for you Paul, I think you should go. It's just what you need to get your confidence back."

Arrangements were made to ensure I had the medication I needed for the trip's length, and I was thoroughly checked out by doctors. I got the green light – I could go.

I saw this as a true Godsend. I would be working hard and all day long, but that's just what I needed to keep me sober and off drugs, and to get my mojo back as Dr. Keroic said. Just knowing that somebody wanted my services again really boosted my confidence, and I knew that doing broadcast work again would only help me feel better about myself.

The last thing I had to do was tell my children what I was about to do. Their reaction wasn't at all like mine to this piece of news.

In fact, they basically went ballistic on me.

◽ ◽ ◽

I can't say that I blame how my children reacted to the news that I was heading right back into the same kind of work that I was doing before my suicide attempt.

There was one thing I knew for sure about my life, and that was that my children loved me and cared about me. It was because they cared so much about me that they basically had a total meltdown on me when I told them I was going to go to the Czech Republic to help broadcast the sledge hockey world championships.

They were convinced I needed more time to recuperate. They felt that the way I was living was what led to my suicide attempt, and that by going back to the same thing would result in a relapse for me. They thought that as soon as I got out of the country and away from doctors, I would stop taking my medication and start drinking again and using drugs.

I understood how they felt. I really did. And I understood that they were yelling at me because they cared for me and didn't want me to relapse.

I truly understood how they felt, but I did not agree.

Being able to do broadcasting work, playing sledge hockey, doing motivational talks…those things did not lead to my downfall. It was alcohol and drugs that led to my downfall.

My future was very uncertain for me, but there was one thing I was certain about. I was never going to put another drug in my body again, or ever start drinking again. But they didn't believe my oath I guess, and they were still feeling the intense hurt after what I had done just two months prior.

I knew where they were coming from. It was hard to tell them that I was going regardless how they felt about it, but in my mind I wanted to go. I felt that I almost had to go in fact, to get back to doing the things that I loved to do.

This trip wasn't going to lead to a relapse. It was going to lead to a re-start to a better life for me. However they disagreed – completely.

Nikki was especially adamant, telling me I was going to go back to being the "big shit" again and then relapse into drinking and drugs again. She had been especially hurt by what I had done and told me I had lived a lie my whole life – and now here I was, heading back down the same path.

However I just knew that wasn't going to be the case. So despite my daughters pleading with me not to go, I went. On April 23 I flew to the Czech Republic with the blessing of my doctors, but not the blessing of my daughters.

Stephanie eventually came around and forgave me for making the trip. She basically forgave me for everything. Nikki did not.

It's my hope that Nikki will find a way to forgive me one day too. But getting back to doing something productive was something I felt I just had to do, and that's what I did.

I just had to take advantage of this opportunity to try and live properly once again.

▫ ▫ ▫

Everything happens for a reason, or so many people say. I guess it does, but trying to figure out the reason things happen sometimes can be tough.

However I think I knew right away the reason that I got that unexpected phone call from the IPC offering me work as a broadcaster.

The reason was – I was being offered a second chance to do things right.

I assured my daughters that things would be different. In retrospect that wasn't the right thing to do. What I should have focused on saying to them was that I was going to be different. What I was doing for a living wasn't what was causing me such pain; it was HOW I was living that caused me pain, along with my substance abuse.

I understood that now. My jobs weren't the problem. I was the problem.

Maybe some people can be social drinkers, or recreational drug users. I am not one of them.

From the time the police came to get me in my apartment the night I attempted suicide, I started to realize how foolish I had been with my habits.

I could have easily died that night. How could have I sunk so low, trying to take my own life?

It was because of the drugs and alcohol. Even saying that is blaming the drugs and alcohol instead of myself so let me rephrase that – it was because of what I became when using drugs and alcohol.

As soon as I checked into the psych ward, I made a vow – I was never going to drink or put any drugs into my body again. I knew I had been given a second chance at life and the only way to take advantage of that properly was to abstain permanently.

I believed I would do it. The bottom line was that my daughters didn't believe me. They saw this trip so soon after my suicide attempt as a danger to relapse; I saw it as an opportunity to stay clean.

Off I went to the Czech Republic despite what they saw.

From the moment I got there I felt overwhelming happiness. I wasn't just happy, I was ecstatic.

In the time I was there, I honestly felt better than I had felt at any other time in my life. It was like I was completely renewed.

By the time the tournament started I was now three months clean and sober, and healthier than I'd been in decades thanks to the care provided to me by the doctors and my family during my rehab. I was so happy just to be alive that every moment of that trip was like a fresh new adventure.

Man did I work on that trip though! They wanted me to do every game, day and night, and I did every game day and night. That was just what I needed. I didn't have a lot of time to sit down and think, or even more importantly, sit down and drink. I was never tempted once to go back to my old way of living while I was there and I haven't since.

The great goalie Dominik Hasek, a hero in his homeland of the Czech Republic, was there and I got to spend some time and get to know him during the tournament. The games were excellent, and my focus was sharp when I was doing the color. Anyone's focus is better when your body is free of drugs.

I had always loved broadcasting and whenever I was doing games, I was always pumped up and happy. But things were different now. Free from the grips of addiction for the first time in my life, I was pumped up and happy all the time, not just when I was broadcasting. Being there was a real joy for me and a clear sign that I would be able to bounce back and live a better life than the one I had been living.

While I was there I also got a chance to go and visit Auschwitz, which is something I will never forget for the rest of my life.

On a rare off day at the tournament, there was someone who wanted to go and see the memorial to the concentration camp survivors. It is very close to the Czech border and when I was asked if I wanted to come along, I jumped at the opportunity.

In 2009 I was also close to Auschwitz at another tournament, but never made it over. It was a second chance to go (I seemed to be getting a lot of those recently), and we drove across the border and spent several hours there.

It was incredibly moving. It's impossible to describe all of the emotions one gets when being inside the place where there was such a horrific experience that took place; the day was rewarding, devastating and uplifting all at the same time. I know that doesn't make sense to some people, but that's the range of feelings one goes through when walking through Auschwitz.

Every Jewish person should go to Auschwitz if they get the chance. I am glad I did, as being there was one of the greatest experiences of my life in ways I can't properly express.

And it is also difficult to express how much that trip meant to me overall; just to be back working and free of drugs. Even when things were going well for me in the past, I always had something to complain about, or acted in egotistical and selfish ways, or never had any contentment. That wasn't the case this time.

This time was different. This time I saw the world without the fog of drugs clouding my brain. It was the happiest seven days of my life.

❏ ❏ ❏

I came back home revitalized. I guess Stephanie saw what the trip had meant to me right away, because she came around and warmed back up to me immediately. Nikki was a different story as I said, but I was still glad I went.

I was also glad I was back home at Stephanie's house, where I wound up staying until September of 2019. Those next five months were important to my healing. I went right back to Dr. Keroic when I returned and got right back involved with all the various programs they were offering.

I continued to volunteer for any additional programs they had to make me stronger mentally. I kept taking my medications, but I was being slowly weaned off of them. I was living a clean and sober lifestyle and seeing the world without drugs lingering in my system for the first time in decades.

I was involved in AA and eating healthy. It is amazing what can come into your life when you escape being a drug addict. I had been at the absolute bottom emotionally on January 30, 2019 but now I was able to appreciate my life more thanks to finally having seen the light about what drugs and alcohol were doing to my body and mind.

It was so liberating for me. I still had concerns about the future, about what I was going to do to keep working on a regular basis. I still had my long term health concerns and other worries to deal with. But I now looked at my life with a fresh set of eyes and was able to focus on the moment and enjoy my life more for what it was.

After all those years of telling people to never give up, to fight through adversity, to be strong – I was finally able to take my own advice.

I was now giving myself the kind of love that I had tried to give to other people through my speeches and talks. I was no longer living a lie I was practicing what I preached.

CHAPTER 33

GOUCHE LIVE

One of my best friends in the world is Kerry Goulet. "Gouche" and I met just before the 2006 Olympics in Torino. Kerry was helping to run an event for the terrific charity "Shoot for a Cure" that raises funds for spinal cord injuries, headed by Barry Monroe, and I was one of the celebrities asked to be at the event.

He was also at the event at Downsview Park in 2007 where my gold medal was stolen from me (which you read about earlier). He was working with his "Stop Concussions" charity, and we became very, very close after that, as he was really helpful to me during that frantic time.

I eventually became an Ambassador for Stop Concussions and through that association, had the opportunity to travel with him to Austria, Germany and basically all around the world helping to promote that great cause. We've had many great times together over the years.

Stop Concussions is such an important initiative. I've filled in giving talks for them several times over the years, as Kerry and former NHLer Keith Primeau do such important work helping make sports safer for everyone. I became so involved that in 2011 I actually became the first Paralympic athlete to donate my brain after I die to Boston University for their research into brain trauma that comes as the result of being an athlete.

Kerry has always been there for me, he's been a truly great friend. He and his wife Toni were both there when I woke up in the psych ward after my attempted suicide. I will never forget Kerry's standing by me at my darkest hour; he is a true friend indeed.

We had kicked around the idea of maybe doing a show together for a few years, and in November, 2019, that idea became a reality.

Graeme Rouston of The Hockey News approached us and asked us if we'd be interested in providing some content under their label (along with the Sports Illustrated brand), and we jumped at the chance to work together.

We started doing the shows at The Hockey News offices, but when COVID hit us (more about that later), we had to do it virtually as their offices closed down.

That didn't stop us, however, as we did our "Gouche Live with Paul Rosen" shows daily at 4 pm, Monday to Friday, and at 7 pm on Mondays.

The Monday shows were especially important to the both of us. "Mental Health Monday shows" explore issues directly relating to mental health issues, which for obvious reasons (as you've just read) are vitally important to me.

They are important to Kerry too. Kerry's sister Karen passed away last year after a long struggle with alcohol abuse and her death was directly related to that. We feel it's so important to do what we can to help others who are facing the mental health challenges that Karen and I – and to some extent all of us – face on a daily basis.

We did more than 400 shows, and it became a big part of my life. It's an amazing amount of fun but like most independently produced shows, you don't do them for the money you do them for the fun. Getting to do something I truly enjoy with a person I consider to be one of my best friends was just priceless to me, however.

I branched out and started doing my own show, "The Rosen Report" in 2021 and that too has been a great deal of fun. We do shows Tuesday, Thursday and Saturday and I am so grateful to be able to talk sports, something I really love to do.

I get a chance to talk sports with a lot of truly great people and we've had some amazing guests on since we started it. Hearing their great stories and talking about what's happening in the sports world today on a regular basis is a great thrill for me, and I'm enjoying every moment of The Rosen Report, especially interacting with our great audience.

That's what life is all about for me now. Enjoying every moment I can, doing the things I like to do, with the people that I want to do them with. Being involved in these types of shows with Kerry allowed me to do just that.

None of us knows what the future will bring, but if we can find ways to enjoy the present, the future will take care of itself.

Thank you Kerry…thanks for everything.

CHAPTER 34

BATTLING COVID

I started 2020 feeling really good. There would be some sledge hockey events for me to cover later in the year, and I knew that my motivational speaking would take on an even more impactful meaning because of what had happened to me.

Attempting suicide was a source of shame at first, but I learned through my therapy that it could also be a source of hope for other people. It had now been a year since that awful night, but I have demonstrated that recovery is possible if you are willing to let go of the past, be honest with others and yourself, and be open to accepting help.

I was eternally grateful for the second chance I was being given, so I looked forward to the future and was living every day to the fullest.

On February 4, 2020, I received my One Year Medallion from AA. That was a very proud moment for me. It truly is one day at a time, and that is how I am taking it. But my vow of sobriety is forever in my mind, and I knew with the help and support I was getting I'd make it.

I also know that I can still help and support other people to make it too. My plan was to get back into work in the spring and look for all opportunities to contribute to helping people wherever I could.

The darkness had lifted and the light had come for me. I had a real bounce in my step as I made plans to get a place of my own sometime soon and spend all the time I could with my new girlfriend Arianna.

I met her in the summer of 2019 and it was love at first site for both of us. Arianna is such a tremendous soul and beautiful both inside and out. But finding love with her really helped me recover from my trauma, and we spent all the time we could together.

She's much younger than I am (she was 24 and I was 59 when we first met), so my family was pretty shocked when I first told them about her. But she became a part of our family quickly, as they all saw what I saw in her – just a beautiful person who was so good for me to be around.

Thanks in large part to Arianna, I was happier than I had been in decades.

Gouche Live featuring Paul Rosen was doing quite well and we were having a blast doing the show at the Hockey News studios. I was staying busy and looking forward to a productive and healthy year.

Then COVID arrived.

We are all suffering through this pandemic to some degree. It's not an easy time for any of us, but it's especially difficult for people who depend on crowds gathering for a living, and for those of us who are recovering addicts. Meeting together in groups to help us keep getting through that adversity is an important part of AA.

I fall into both groups of course. Like many of us, trying to navigate through a pandemic has been one of the greatest challenges of my life. It's hard enough being in recovery at the best of times, but it's especially challenging in a pandemic. For more than a year, I haven't been able to attend an in-person therapy session with AA, or attend any other group programs as they've all been put on hold.

My broadcasting work was suspended as well, as all sledge hockey events were shuttered along with a great deal of other sporting events. There have been no calls to be a speaker to schools or anywhere else in times like these, so that work is on hold as well. We're still doing The Rosen Report and some shows with Kerry Goulet, but it's all virtual now as we try and navigate through the challenges of doing that.

Everybody is going through this; the whole world is affected by COVID. However for some people, it's not nearly as bad as it is for others. If you have a steady office job but can work from home, it may be inconvenient but you are still doing OK financially. Just imagine how difficult it is for front line care workers, or those that have lost their jobs, or those that have no family or safe home to retreat to until things open up again.

If COVID had come along before my recovery started, there's a very strong chance I wouldn't be alive today. I wouldn't have been mentally strong enough to face the personal challenges I faced because of the pandemic.

NEVER GIVE UP

I still stay in touch with my AA sponsor. I still have virtual talks from time to time. And I had Arianna in my life, who was a true Godsend for me. We will get through this together and come out of it much stronger on the other side as a result.

I am so fortunate to have a man named Jimmy Avrams in my life as well. When hard times hit in your life, you find out who your friends are in a hurry and Jimmy has always been there for me. We've known each other since we were 17 years of age, a lifetime ago.

Jimmy and I have been close friends for decades and I can't thank him enough for all he has done for me over the years, through good times and bad. When I needed a place to stay, he welcomed me into his home with open arms. He is a true friend in every sense of the word, and I love you Jimmy.

Life can be hard at times – very hard actually as you've seen with my story – but it's made so much better by having people like Arianna and Jimmy with me every step of the way.

Notice the change in my tone from the story of my earlier years? It's very different. That's because I am very different. There have been no drugs or alcohol in my body for more than two years and there won't be again. I can now clearly see that life really is all in how you look at it, and you need clear eyes to see it properly. That's not possible when they are clouded by substance abuse.

As I write this, every indication is that the end of the pandemic is near. A time will come very soon that events will return, sports will return and we'll all get back to normal, or at least very close to it. I along with all of us look forward to that day very much.

I will continue to dedicate my life to helping others now and in the future. Everything I have gone through has made me a better and stronger person.

So that's pretty much my life story up until early 2021. I am very grateful I was able to get it all down on paper and share it with you. Thank you for reading it.

Now to conclude this book, I would like to share with you something very important. This is a question that I had to answer during my comeback from my suicide attempt, and a question we should all think about deeply and answer for ourselves.

That question is – what is the meaning of my life?

CHAPTER 35

FOUR STORIES

I have been honest throughout this book. It's been painfully honest at times, as I want the record of my life to be clear and transparent. It's my hope that perhaps someone reads this and comes to realize that how happy they are is really up to them, not dependent on what happens to them.

It took me a long while to discover that and really live it. Now I hope to live that philosophy the rest of my life, for however long that lasts.

What's the meaning of my life? Boy – that's a question I asked myself while I was putting these memoirs together with my friend Roger Lajoie many times.

I'm going to include a few stories here now that will illustrate what I believe the meaning of my life is. Thinking about them again gave me the answer to my question, as I realized I had more value to people than I often thought.

You should always be kind. You never know what a good-hearted gesture will mean to someone else…as these stories will show you.

▫ ▫ ▫

By 2001, I had the chance to meet and know a lot of great people in the sports world as a result of my time with Team Canada. It was a real thrill for me to have the opportunity to meet and mingle with some great names in the sports world, believe me.

Many of these athletes were so kind and generous with their time. One person right at the top of that list was Joe Sakic.

As much as I enjoyed meeting people like the Colorado Avalanche's great superstar, what brought me even more joy was when I could introduce people like Joe Sakic to other people, so they could experience that thrill of meeting a famous person as well.

Sakic is just a tremendous person. I cannot say enough good things about him. And thanks to Joe's kindness and generosity, I had a chance to bring my great friend Shayne Smith to Detroit in 2001 for a memory he will never forget…and neither will I.

You will remember from earlier in the book that Shayne was the young man that introduced me to sled hockey in the first place. Without him, none of what happened to me on the ice over the years would have been possible, so I was looking for a small way to try and thank him.

I came up with a plan and it wouldn't have been possible without Sakic's co-operation. Shayne loved Joe Sakic, so I contacted Joe and he arranged for great seats for when the Avalanche were playing the Detroit Red Wings at Joe Louis Arena.

I didn't tell Shayne anything about it. I just told him I was going to pick him up and take him somewhere, not letting on what I had in mind.

I talked about Shayne earlier, but let me say again – what a sensational kid he was and what a great young man he's turned out to be, despite being a triple amputee.

We drove all the way to Detroit, and he was delighted to see that we were going to see an NHL game at The Joe. But that was the least of it. Thanks to Sakic, it was pre-arranged that we would get to go into the Avalanche dressing room and meet the players before the game.

The look on Shayne's face was priceless. There, standing in the center of the room, was one of his heroes in Joe Sakic. He couldn't believe it, what a thrill for him. The tears flowed that day friends, and it wasn't just Shayne who was crying. All the players, including Sakic, were emotional too as they saw what it meant for a young man who had overcame so much to get the chance to be in an NHL dressing room with all of those great stars.

I will never forget that day for the rest of my life. Shayne won't either, but the joy I experienced in just seeing how happy it made him was worth the drive and the work to get it all organized. I really learned that day what you do for yourself can bring you joy, but nothing beats the joy you experience when you can do something for someone else.

Now Shayne is all grown, and he was even in Tokyo, Japan for the wheelchair rugby event in the 2021 Paralympics. I am so proud of him and happy for him!

Thank you so much Joe Sakic…and thank you Shayne. That trip to Detroit was the least I could have done for all you did for me, but that day means more to ME than you'll ever know.

◘ ◘ ◘

It's 2003. By now I've been to the Olympics and my national profile has led me to be asked to do many speaking events. I am doing an event one day which is being covered by the Barrie Examiner.

After it's over, I was interviewed for a story that the paper was doing on me. It was a nice polite interview, but I could sense that the reporter asking me the questions wanted to ask me something that she didn't want to include in the newspaper story to follow.

We conclude the interview and it turns out I was right. The reporter wanted to know if I ever spoke to people individually to help them through their own tough times, or did I just do talks for larger audiences.

I told her I try and help everyone I can and quite often will make some time to speak to someone privately. It was then that she told me about her father.

She told me her father was in the hospital in Newmarket. He was 73 years old. Due to illness he had to have both of his legs amputated. He was angry and depressed by what had happened to him.

The reporter didn't have to ask me twice; this was the kind of thing I welcomed doing. I was making a few bucks doing my talks for schools, business and other community groups, but I was always happy to try and encourage people privately at no charge. I never wanted a cent for that; I just felt it was the right thing for me to do.

I had bounced back from losing a limb and the amputation had actually made my life better. A lot of people were encouraged by what I had done. I got the address of the hospital and arranged to come and see him.

I walk in. He has two daughters and one granddaughter there. I smile and introduce myself to him, hoping I can encourage him to feel better about things.

I won't get into the specifics from that first meeting, but he was really rude to me. There was no getting through to him that day, so I turned around and left.

His daughter apologized profusely and thanked me for coming anyway.

"That's OK," I told her. "I'll try again."

So I did. Despite him basically tossing me out of the room the first time, I did go back a second time. The second reception wasn't much better than the first.

This time, however, at least he was talking more. So I just let him talk. People think I do a great job encouraging people by my talking, but what most people want you to do is just listen to them.

I listened to him rant. He wanted to kill himself. He felt his life was over and he saw no future for himself now that he had lost both his legs.

Everybody needs to be talked to in a different way when they are going terrible situations like he was. I felt he needed some tough love.

I told him if he killed himself, not only would he die but his entire family would suffer because of it. I told him to imagine the guilt they would feel. I told him to think of his youngest granddaughter who was just 15 years old.

I asked him to consider how she would feel, and what she might possibly do, if he did the unthinkable and killed himself. Would that lead her to thinking that suicide is OK, I asked him? How would you feel if as a result of you killing yourself, I told him, she might consider it all right to kill herself if something bad happened to her?

Harsh words, I know – but I knew I had to reach him and reach him quickly. Those words made him take the focus off of himself and put it on the people in his life. If you can't find a way to live for yourself, then find a way to live for your family (those thoughts helped ME stay alive many times over the years as you've already read).

That got through to him. With tears in his eyes he actually thanked me, and we had a terrific talk. He was soon able to leave the hospital and when he did, he left in a much better frame of mind.

We became quite good friends. Impulsively one day I even gave him my Team Canada jersey from the 2002 Paralympics as a gift to encourage him that life really could go on after amputation. I treasured that jersey, but I figured he needed more than I did at that point so I was pleased to give it to him. He was absolutely thrilled.

We stayed in touch and despite the serious health challenges that went along with his amputation, he never considered suicide again. He was able to spend his last few years in peace and in the company of his loving family.

In 2005 he passed away. I was asked to come to the funeral and I did. His children and granddaughters were there, and the youngest granddaughter came up and thanked me profusely for what I had done for her grandfather.

"You helped make his last few years so much better," she said.

I never know what to say when somebody says that to me, as I've been blessed to hear that a few times in my life. I really was choked up, so I just hugged her and went to pay my respects to her grandfather.

I've often been asked if I kept any mementoes from my playing days. I have several actually; masks, sticks, pucks, my medals, a few jerseys.

But my jersey from the 2002 Paralympics I gave away, and I am so glad that I did.

* * *

It's 2009. By now I've been to two Olympics and won a gold medal. My speaking career has really taken off and I'm doing a lot of motivational talks.

I am speaking to a group of students at Malvern High School in Scarborough one morning. My talk to them is about the importance of having positive role models in your life. I said to the kids that their role models should come from people they know and respect personally, instead of making athletes and entertainers you've never even met your role models.

My talk is well received and the kids give me a big hand. That in itself was quite an accomplishment, as this school had some really rough students – or so I was told.

I've always believed, however, there are no bad kids. There are just bad parents or bad circumstances kids have had to deal with. I enjoy talking to all sorts of groups, but being able to speak to younger people is a great pleasure for me. Kids are more prone to listen to you and learn if you take the time with them.

One young man had a lot to say about my talk on having role models, wearing his ball cap backwards and low hanging jeans.

"Kobe Bryant is my role model," he said during my talk. "I've never met him."

Despite his somewhat ragged appearance, I could sense that this was an incredible kid. He just had something about him; you could see it in his eyes.

I told him that there was nothing wrong with admiring Kobe Bryant or any other famous person, but he should find someone he knew personally to be his role model. I repeated that it was important to have role models you knew and could talk to instead of famous people you had never met.

I was holding onto my gold medal from the Olympics while he was talking. He was looking at it then he looked up at me.

"Would you be my role model then?" he said." I know you now."

I gave that kid a big smile and told him that it would be an honor for me to be his role model. That got him to smile in return. We stayed in touch a bit over the years, as I tried to offer him encouragement as he found his way through school and through life.

Three years later that young man, who the teachers told me had been struggling in high school, called to let me know that he had just been accepted at university and was on his way.

Every child is born with the potential to do great things. That potential just needs to be allowed to develop. One day that young man is going to be a role model himself, and I could not be happier for him.

◻ ◻ ◻

It's 2015. As you've already read this was a pretty low period for me personally. But I was still a popular speaker at schools and was doing a lot of talks in front of students.

I was feeling pretty shitty, but if I could get some kids to feel better by talking to them, then it really helped them.

And it really helped me – who is kidding who here.

My talk on this day was at Bialik Hebrew Day School, a Jewish school for grades one through six. What a charming group these kids were. I really enjoyed my chance to speak with them that day.

After I was done, the principal of the school came over to thank me profusely for being there. He said he had never seen the kids in the school so quiet when somebody was talking to them. He told me I had really gotten their attention.

NEVER GIVE UP

I smiled and said thanks. I told him how much I enjoyed coming to schools and let him know that his kids were great. While we were talking, I looked over my shoulder and saw a young girl who I later found out was in Grade 3. She was standing off to the side, smiling, and it looked like she wanted to talk to me.

"Hi there!" I said to her and motioned for her to come over. Shyly she did.

She looked up into my face and said "Rosey I love you" and gave me a hug.

I've had some wonderful interactions with people after I've done a talk, but that might have been the best one of all time! I had tears of joy as I hugged her back. "I love you too!" I said.

A nice looking woman then came up to us with a huge smile on her face. She had no right arm.

She introduced herself. She was the young girl's mother. She had lost her arm to cancer. When she found out that I would be speaking at the school, she made sure she and her daughter would be there to hear me speak.

I thanked her so much for coming and told her I hope that my talk gave her some encouragement. What she said next really surprised me.

"I am doing fine Rosey thank you. But I didn't come for me, I came for my daughter."

As it turns out, she had recuperated well both mentally and physically from losing her limb…but her daughter had not. Seeing her Mom without an arm had devastated her daughter emotionally and as a result, she had pulled away from her mother.

"I watched my daughter's face every second you were speaking," she continued. "She couldn't take her eyes off you and listened to every word you said. When you were finished speaking she finally looked over at me and smiled at me for the first time in months.

"Mr. Rosen, I think this talk you gave may have brought me back my daughter."

That left me speechless (there's a first time for everything I know!). I didn't know what to say.

I gave them my number and shortly afterwards I went over to their house to have dinner with them. Her mother was right – her daughter had completely turned around. She was constantly playing and smiling with her Mom. You could see the love shared between them every time they looked at each other.

I was so incredibly touched by the whole thing driving home that night. The smile on my face I got from seeing their happiness must have stayed with me for days.

You can make a difference in somebody's life sometimes just by saying a few positive words of encouragement. It may not seem like it's a big deal when you do, but you never know the impact some encouraging words can make on a person.

Always be quick to offer a kind word. If you ever get to see the impact it can make, you'll know why. I certainly did that night.

□ □ □

Those stories brought back some touching memories for me. I have many more stories too, as I've been blessed to have had many touching moments like these happen to me over the years – but I'll stop with those four.

I don't include these stories to make myself out to be a hero. I include them to show you how much I was affected by the way I somehow managed to affect other people with my motivational talks over the years.

Even at times where I was struggling badly myself, I was able to help others alleviate the pain they were feeling. So many times in my life I felt worthless, but so many times I was able to help others find their worth.

I obviously have some kind of a gift with the way I am able to reach people with my talks. My message really resonates with many people and I was able to help them.

Mental health, as I found out first hand, can turn on dime. What we say to each other can make such a difference.

I want to conclude this book now by finally answering the question I have been trying to answer for many years.

That question again is – what is the meaning of my life?

CHAPTER 36

LIFE'S MEANING

It is an incredibly difficult task to sit down and put your life story down on paper. In my case it was also very painful to go over the details and talk as frankly as I have in these pages about the mistakes I've made in my life. I made so many mistakes. I will spend the rest of my life trying to correct them and be a better person.

I look back at my journey and I shake my head. My life has certainly been an interesting one, and that is an understatement.

I come from a humble background, so having had the opportunity to have played in three Paralympics, three world championships, three World Cups and to have worn the Team Canada jersey in international competition so many times, was pretty amazing when you think about.

To have had the chance to be a broadcaster with the CBC and TSN was certainly a thrill for a guy who never went to journalism school or had any training in that field. Just being able to do that was also incredible.

My motivational speaking career was one I cherished as well. To have the responsibility – and it is a true responsibility – to speak to others and to try and help them feel motivated to have a better life is an incredible honor. The level of trust that a school, an organization or business shows in you to allow you to do that is very flattering. I am deeply grateful.

But as you've read in these pages, I often found it difficult to live my own life the way I was telling other people to live theirs. I couldn't seem to be able to follow my own advice.

Even at the best of times in my life (and maybe ESPECIALLY at the best of times in my life), I sabotaged my own happiness by acting terribly towards other people. I look back at some of my actions now, especially things I did to my family and my Team Canada teammates, and I'm embarrassed to remember what I did.

The drugs and alcohol were a big influence on my behavior, but the responsibility for my mistakes is mine to bear. I accept it.

I have apologized to everyone I've hurt over the years. I'm now trying to live my best life in the time I have left on this planet and make up for the mistakes I made when I was younger. It was therapeutic for me in a way to write this book. Getting it all down on paper helped me.

As I write this, I'm 61 years old. We are just getting through a devastating pandemic that has hurt all of us emotionally and financially. It was especially a very difficult time for me, as my income slipped to basically zero and I couldn't access the usual treatments and services I was using as a recovering alcoholic and drug abuser.

But I survived the worst of the pandemic, as most of us have, and thank God for that. There are better days ahead for all of us. We live to fight another day.

And of course, I must always live with the ultimate mistake I made on January 30, 2019. That was the night I did what I tell everyone not to do – I gave up. I gave up on myself and I gave up on my life. I attempted suicide.

It is now almost three years since that horrible night. I am clean and sober, I feel better than I have in decades, and I am finally at peace.

So you might be saying to yourself – come on Rosey, answer the question you said you were going to answer. What is the meaning of your life? What is the meaning behind your suicide attempt? What is the meaning behind this wild ride of a life you have just shared with us?!

Let me finally tell you what it is.

It took me a while to come up with the answer, but I did. It really started to come to me when I made that visit to Auschwitz in April 2019 that I told you about a few pages back.

We all want to find meaning in our lives. We all want to understand why things happen. Going to Auschwitz was a real eye opener for me. That trip was the start of me getting my answer.

What was the meaning of Auschwitz, I remember asking myself as I walked around it? What possible meaning could come from horrors like what had happened there?

In his book Man's Search for Meaning, Viktor Frankl (an Auschwitz survivor), describes how he and others survived his time in the concentration camp. They survived because they put the needs of others ahead of their own. If they had only one piece of bread, those who shared the meager portion with others were the ones that made it through.

Frankl often quoted Nietzsche: "He who has a why to live for can bear almost any how." The prisoners who held on to their "why" were the ones who made it through the horrible ordeal they were all facing.

"Everything can be taken from a man but one thing: the last of the human freedoms—to choose one's attitude in any given set of circumstances, to choose one's own way." What a great Frankl quote that is. And that's what those survivors were doing – they were choosing their own attitude and their own way. They were choosing to live so others could live.

I left Auschwitz a changed man. I said earlier that every Jewish person should visit there, I'll amend that – every human being should visit there.

I became very interested in Frankl's work after my visit to Auschwitz and Roger recommending his books to me. The exercise of writing my book really got me to think about the meaning of my life, in the same way Frankl studied the meaning of all life.

Frankl gave us quotes to think about like these:

> *"For the meaning of life differs from man to man, from day to day and from hour to hour. What matters, therefore, is not the meaning of life in general but rather the specific meaning of a person's life at a given moment."*

> *"One should not search for an abstract meaning of life. Everyone has his own specific vocation or mission in life to carry out a concrete assignment which demands fulfillment. Therein he cannot be replaced, nor can his life be repeated. Thus, everyone's task is as unique as is his specific opportunity to implement it."*

Those words really resonated with me. It really got me to thinking what was the point of everything I went through, what meaning could I take from all of it?

Frankl also wrestled with this question. He was finally challenged by a student one day to specifically say what the meaning of HIS life was. He searched for his own answer, and eventually came up with the quote you first saw at the start of this book.

"The meaning of my life is to help others find the meaning of theirs." – Viktor Frankl

That is my answer as well. The meaning of Paul Rosen's life is to help other people find the meaning of theirs. The meaning of my suicide attempt is therefore this:

I tried to kill myself so you won't.

◘ ◘ ◘

I will still do motivational talks whenever I can. I will always try and encourage people to hang in there. I tell great stories and have a bit of a gift in the entertaining way that I tell them. I am very grateful for that.

Sometimes I'm questioned as to why I can be so good at helping other people when I couldn't help myself. I'm also asked how I could have possibly tried to kill myself after having helped so many others not give up on their lives.

Great questions…here's the answer to them.

Many times after my talks someone would come up to me and say something like "Great chat Rosey, but you don't know what I'm going through." Now I can hand them a copy of this book and smile and say "oh yes I do."

Having attempted suicide doesn't make me less qualified to be a motivational speaker. It makes me MORE qualified to be a motivational speaker.

I went through what I went through in life to help people get through what they are going through in their lives. That is my mission. That is the meaning of my life…to help you find the meaning of yours.

If you are feeling suicidal, please reach out for help. You can email me directly at info@paulrosen.ca. I guarantee you I will respond. There are many other sources of help out there for you as well that you can use. All you have to do is Google and you'll find multiple sources of assistance available in the community in which you live. There are many qualified people out there who can assist you in your darkest times.

We have come a long way in eliminating the stigma attached to mental health. Do not be ashamed to ask for help like I was in January, 2019.

If you are struggling with addictions to drugs and/or alcohol, contact Alcoholics Anonymous. They can help you. I know that first hand. They are amazing people who can help you break free from your addictions. Give them a chance to help you if you think you need it.

Life is good even in its worst moments. It was a lesson I needed to learn and I have finally learned it. There is always hope for a better day tomorrow.

> **My friends please hear this and believe this – when you have to go through hell in order to climb back up to the top of the mountain, it can be devastating. But once you get through it and reach the mountain top again – the view is spectacular. When you suffer greatly, the end of the suffering will provide you with a view of life that is breath taking. It is worth the struggle. Please believe that.**

In the time I have left on this planet I will continue to help others through my motivational talks. I will continue to try and be a better person, a better father and a better friend. After putting all these words onto paper, I now know my life and everything that happened in it does have meaning…all of the good and all of the bad too.

The meaning of my life is to help you find the meaning of yours. Thank you so much for reading my story and I hope to be able to meet many of you in person down the road.

God bless you and your families. Go out there and live the best life you can every day.

And please remember….

Never Give Up.

Paul Rosen

September 1, 2021

ABOUT THE AUTHOR

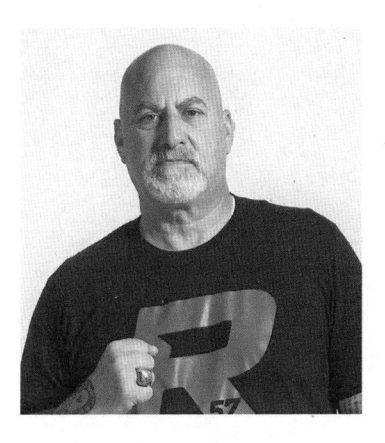

Paul Rosen is one of the greatest goalies in the history of the Paralympics. After overcoming the loss of his leg, he was a star in goal for Team Canada for more than a decade in numerous Olympic Games and world championships, posting incredible goaltending records. He later became a noted broadcaster with several major news organizations including TSN and the CBC, and a well-known public speaker and leading advocate for mental health, especially during his many talks to children in schools across the country. He has hosted numerous podcasts in the past several years, and has used his platform many times to talk about his experiences and how he can help others battle through their adversities. He has spent many years encouraging people to "Never Give Up!" and to find the meaning of their lives while discovering the meaning of his own. This is his first book. You can visit him at www.paulrosen.ca.

Roger Lajoie has been a sports writer, broadcaster and hockey executive for more than four decades. Among his four previous books were "The Goal of My Life" with legendary Canadian hockey hero Paul Henderson (a Globe and Mail bestseller) and "The Road to Hockeytown" with Jimmy Devellano. You can visit him at www.rogerlajoie.com.

Printed in Canada